a LANGE medical book

Vander's Renal Physiology

Sixth Edition

Douglas C. Eaton, PhD

*Distinguished Professor of Physiology
and Professor of Pediatrics
Emory University School of Medicine
Atlanta, Georgia*

John P. Pooler, PhD

*Associate Professor of Physiology
Emory University School of Medicine
Atlanta, Georgia*

Lange Medical Books/McGraw-Hill
Medical Publishing Division

New York   Chicago   San Francisco   Lisbon   London   Madrid   Mexico City
Milan   New Delhi   San Juan   Seoul   Singapore   Sydney   Toronto

Vander's Renal Physiology, Sixth Edition

1 2 3 4 5 6 7 8 9 0 DOCDOC 0 9 8 7 6 5 4

ISSN: 1548-338X
ISBN: 0-07-135728-9

Notice

Medicine is an ever-changing science. As new research and clinical experience broaden our knowledge, changes in treatment and drug therapy are required. The authors and the publisher of this work have checked with sources believed to be reliable in their efforts to provide information that is complete and generally in accord with the standards accepted at the time of publication. However, in view of the possibility of human error or changes in medical sciences, neither the authors nor the publisher nor any other party who has been involved in the preparation or publication of this work warrants that the information contained herein is in every respect accurate or complete, and they disclaim all responsibility for any errors or omissions or for the results obtained from use of the information contained in this work. Readers are encouraged to confirm the information contained herein with other sources. For example and in particular, readers are advised to check the product information sheet included in the package of each drug they plan to administer to be certain that the information contained in this work is accurate and that changes have not been made in the recommended dose or in the contraindications for administration. This recommendation is of particular importance in connection with new or infrequently used drugs.

This book was set in Adobe Garamond by International Typesetting and Composition.
The editors were Janet Foltin, Harriet Lebowitz, and Regina Y. Brown.
The production supervisor was Catherine H. Saggese.
The text designer was Eve Siegel.
The cover designer was Mary McKeon.
The index was prepared by Herr's Indexing Service.
RR Donnelly was printer and binder.

This book is printed on acid-free paper.

To all our students

Contents

Preface

In this new edition of Arthur Vander's classic text of renal physiology, we set ourselves several goals. The first was to make the text as readable as possible by continuing Dr. Vander's personal, conversational style. We have incorporated into this existing framework changes and additions that reflect recent new knowledge of kidney function.

The second goal was to present as explicitly as possible the interrelationships between blood pressure and renal function, describing how changes in blood pressure generate signals that alter renal excretion of sodium and water, and how renal excretion, by regulating the extracellular fluid volume in the body, ultimately determines blood pressure. Because this is such a complex topic, we of necessity expanded the text description beyond events that are strictly renal in nature.

The third major goal was to exploit our extensive teaching experience to clarify some of the concepts that our students often find troublesome. Unfortunately, the limitations of current knowledge prevent us from clearing up all confusion, specifically in the signaling events that regulate renal function, an area in which we look forward to new developments and insights from the biomedical research community.

To help orient the reader and to prevent students from being mired in details, we added key concepts at the end of each chapter. This feature also highlights the major points throughout the text and allows easy and quick review. We hope that these key concepts, together with the learning objectives, will be effective tools in learning renal physiology.

Renal Functions, Anatomy, and Basic Processes

OBJECTIVES

The student understands the disparate role of the kidneys in maintaining health.

▶ *States the 7 major functions of the kidneys.*

▶ *Defines the balance concept.*

The student understands the structural makeup of the kidneys, their blood supply, and the relation between major functional components.

▶ *Defines the gross structures and their interrelationships: renal pelvis, calyces, renal pyramids, renal medulla (inner and outer zones), renal cortex, papilla.*

▶ *Defines the components of the nephron and their interrelationships: renal corpuscle, glomerulus, nephron, and collecting-duct system.*

▶ *Draws the relationship between glomerulus, Bowman's capsule, and the proximal tubule.*

▶ *Describes the 3 layers separating the lumen of the glomerular capillaries and Bowman's space; defines podocytes, foot processes, and slit diaphragms.*

▶ *Defines glomerular mesangial cells and states their functions and location within the glomerulus.*

▶ *Lists the individual tubular segments in order; states the segments that comprise the proximal tubule, Henle's loop, and the collecting-duct system; defines principal cells and intercalated cells.*

▶ *Lists in order the vessels through which blood flows from the renal artery to the renal vein; contrasts the blood supply to the cortex and the medulla; defines vasa recta and vascular bundles.*

▶ *Describes, in general terms, the differences among superficial cortical, midcortical, and juxtamedullary nephrons.*

▶ *Defines juxtaglomerular apparatus and describes its 3 cell types; states the function of the granular cells.*

The student understands how the 2 kidneys handle substances in order to achieve balance of each.

▶ *Defines the basic renal processes: glomerular filtration, tubular reabsorption, and tubular secretion.*

▶ *Defines renal metabolism of a substance and gives examples.*

The kidneys perform a wide array of functions for the body, most of which are essential for life. Some renal functions have obvious logical and necessary connections to each other. Others seem to be totally independent. Most involve matching renal excretion of substances out of the body to inputs into the body (ie, providing a balance between input and output).

FUNCTIONS

A popular view considers the kidney to be an organ primarily responsible for the removal of metabolic waste from the body. Although this is certainly one function of the kidney, there are other functions that are arguably more important.

Function 1: Regulation of Water and Electrolyte Balance

The balance concept states that our bodies are *in balance* for any substance when the inputs and outputs of that substance are matched. Any difference between input and output leads to an increase or decrease in the amount of a substance within the body. Our input of water and electrolytes is enormously variable and is only sometimes driven in response to body needs. Although we drink water when thirsty, we drink much more because it is a component of beverages that we consume for reasons other than hydration. We also consume food to provide energy, but food often contains large amounts of water. The kidneys respond by varying the output of water in the urine, thereby maintaining balance for water (ie, constant total body water content). Minerals like sodium, potassium, magnesium, and so on are components of foods and generally present far in excess of body needs. As with water, the kidneys excrete minerals at a highly variable rate that, in the aggregate, matches input. One of the amazing feats of the kidneys is their ability to regulate each of these minerals independently (ie, we can be on a high-sodium, low-potassium diet or low-sodium, high-potassium diet, and the kidneys will adjust excretion of each of these substances appropriately[1]).

Function 2: Excretion of Metabolic Waste

Our bodies continuously form end products of metabolic processes. In most cases, those end products serve no function and are harmful at high concentrations. Some of these waste products include urea (from protein), uric acid (from nucleic acids),

---

[1] One point to emphasize, and one that is commonly misunderstood, is that when we have an unusually high or low level of a substance in our body relative to normal, this does not imply that we are perpetually out of balance. To raise the level of a substance in the body, we must be transiently in positive balance. However, once that level reaches a constant value with input and output again equal, we are back in balance. Consider the case of urea, a substance the liver synthesizes continuously. In normal conditions, the kidneys excrete urea at the rate it is synthesized in the body. We are normally *in balance* for urea. If damage to the kidneys occurs, excretion is transiently decreased, and urea accumulates in the body. The higher levels of urea in the blood restore renal urea excretion to its former value despite the damaged kidneys, and we are back in balance even though levels in the body remain high. The same applies to more complex substances, such as acids and bases. When we develop a metabolic acidosis, acid input transiently exceeds acid output. This leads to an accumulation of acids, which, in turn, stimulates renal excretion of acid. Soon excretion matches input (we are back in balance), but there is an elevated amount of acid in the body.

creatinine (from muscle creatine), the end products of hemoglobin breakdown (which give urine much of its color), and the metabolites of various hormones, among many others.

Function 3: Excretion of Bioactive Substances (Hormones and Many Foreign Substances, Specifically Drugs) That Affect Body Function

Physicians have to be mindful of how fast the kidneys excrete drugs in order to prescribe a dose that achieves the appropriate body levels. Hormones in the blood are removed in many ways, mostly in the liver, but a number of hormones are removed in parallel by renal processes.

Function 4: Regulation of Arterial Blood Pressure

Although many people appreciate at least vaguely that the kidneys excrete waste substances like urea (hence the name urine) and salts, few realize the kidneys' crucial role in controlling blood pressure. Blood pressure ultimately depends on blood volume, and the kidneys' maintenance of sodium and water balance achieves regulation of blood volume. Thus, through volume control, the kidneys participate in blood pressure control. They also participate in regulation of blood pressure via the generation of vasoactive substances that regulate smooth muscle in the peripheral vasculature.

Function 5: Regulation of Red Blood Cell Production

Erythropoietin is a peptide hormone that is involved in the control of erythrocyte (red blood cell) production by the bone marrow. Its major source is the kidneys, although the liver also secretes small amounts. The renal cells that secrete it are a particular group of cells in the interstitium. The stimulus for its secretion is a reduction in the partial pressure of oxygen in the kidneys, as occurs, for example, in anemia, arterial hypoxia, and inadequate renal blood flow. Erythropoietin stimulates the bone marrow to increase its production of erythrocytes. Renal disease may result in diminished erythropoietin secretion, and the ensuing decrease in bone marrow activity is one important causal factor of the anemia of chronic renal disease.

Function 6: Regulation of Vitamin D Production

When we think of vitamin D, we often think of sunlight or additives to milk. In vivo vitamin D synthesis involves a series of biochemical transformations, the last of which occurs in the kidneys. The *active* form of vitamin D (1,25-dihydroxyvitamin D_3), is actually made in the kidneys, and its rate of synthesis is regulated by hormones that control calcium and phosphate balance.

Function 7: Gluconeogenesis

Our central nervous system is an obligate user of blood glucose regardless of whether we have just eaten sugary doughnuts or gone without food for a week. Whenever the intake of carbohydrate is stopped for much more than half a day, our body begins to synthesize new glucose (the process of gluconeogenesis) from noncarbohydrate sources (amino acids from protein and glycerol from triglycerides). Most gluconeogenesis occurs in the liver, but a substantial fraction occurs in the kidneys, particularly during a prolonged fast.

Most of what the kidneys actually do to perform the functions just mentioned involves transporting water and solutes between the blood flowing through the kidneys and the lumina of tubules (nephrons and collecting tubules that comprise the working mass of the kidneys). The lumen of a nephron is topologically outside the body, and any substance in the lumen that is not transported back into the blood is eventually excreted in the urine. As we develop renal function in more detail, we constantly refer to tubular structure and the surrounding vasculature. Therefore, in the following section, we present the essential aspects of renal anatomy that are necessary to describe function.

ANATOMY OF THE KIDNEYS AND URINARY SYSTEM

The 2 kidneys lie outside the peritoneal cavity in close apposition to the posterior abdominal wall, 1 on each side of the vertebral column. Each of the 2 kidneys is a bean-shaped structure. The rounded, outer convex surface of each kidney faces the side of the body, and the indented surface, called the *hilum,* is medial. Each hilum is penetrated by a renal artery, renal vein, nerves, and a ureter, which carries urine out of the kidney to the bladder. Each ureter within the kidney is formed from major calyces, which, in turn, are formed from minor calyces. The calyces are funnel-shaped structures that fit over underlying cone-shaped renal tissue called *pyramids.* The tip of each pyramid is called a *papilla* and projects into a minor calyx. The calyces act as collecting cups for the urine formed by the renal tissue in the pyramids. The pyramids are arranged radially around the hilum, with the papillae pointing toward the hilum and the broad bases of the pyramids facing the outside, top, and bottom of the kidney (from the 12-o'clock to the 6-o'clock position). The pyramids constitute the medulla of the kidney. Overlying the medullary tissue is a cortex, and covering the cortical tissue on the very external surface of the kidney is a thin connective tissue capsule (Figure 1–1).

The working tissue mass of both the cortex and medulla is constructed primarily of tubules (nephrons and collecting tubules) and blood vessels (capillaries and capillary-like vessels). Tubules and blood vessels are intertwined or arranged in parallel arrays and, in either case, are always close to each other. Between the tubules and blood vessels lies an *interstitium,* which comprises less than 10% of the renal volume. The interstitium contains scattered interstitial cells (fibroblasts and others) that synthesize an extracellular matrix of collagen, proteoglycans, and glycoproteins.

The cortex and medulla have very different properties structurally and functionally. On closer examination, we see that (1) the cortex has a highly granular appearance, absent in the medulla, and (2) each medullary pyramid is divisible into an outer zone (adjacent to the cortex) and an inner zone, which includes the papilla. All these distinctions reflect the arrangement of the various tubules and blood vessels.

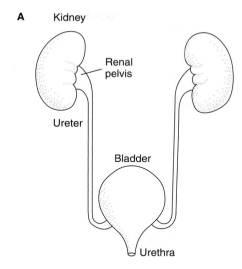

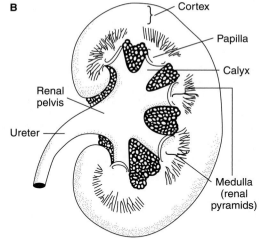

Figure 1–1. **A,** The urinary system. The urine formed by a kidney collects in the renal pelvis and then flows through the ureter into the bladder, from which it is eliminated via the urethra. **B,** Section of a human kidney. Half the kidney has been sliced away. Note that the structure shows regional differences. The outer portion (cortex) contains all the glomeruli. The collecting ducts form a large portion of the inner kidney (medulla), giving it a striped, pyramid-like appearance, and these drain into the renal pelvis. The papilla is in the inner portion of the medulla.

THE NEPHRON

Each kidney contains approximately 1 million *nephrons,* one of which is shown diagrammatically in Figure 1–2. Each nephron consists of a spherical filtering component, called the *renal corpuscle,* and a tubule extending from the renal corpuscle. Let us begin with the renal corpuscle, which is responsible for the initial step in urine formation: the separation of a protein-free filtrate from plasma.

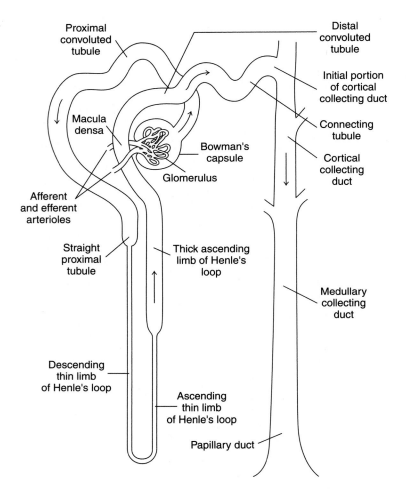

Figure 1–2. Relationships of component parts of a long-looped nephron, which has been "uncoiled" for clarity (relative lengths of the different segments are not drawn to scale). The combination of glomerulus and Bowman's capsule is the renal corpuscle.

The Renal Corpuscle

The renal corpuscle consists of a compact tuft of interconnected capillary loops, the *glomerulus* (pl. *glomeruli*) or glomerular capillaries, surrounded by a balloon-like hollow capsule: Bowman's capsule (Figure 1–3). Blood enters and leaves Bowman's capsule through arterioles that penetrate the surface of the capsule at the vascular pole. A fluid-filled space (the urinary space or Bowman's space) exists within the capsule, and

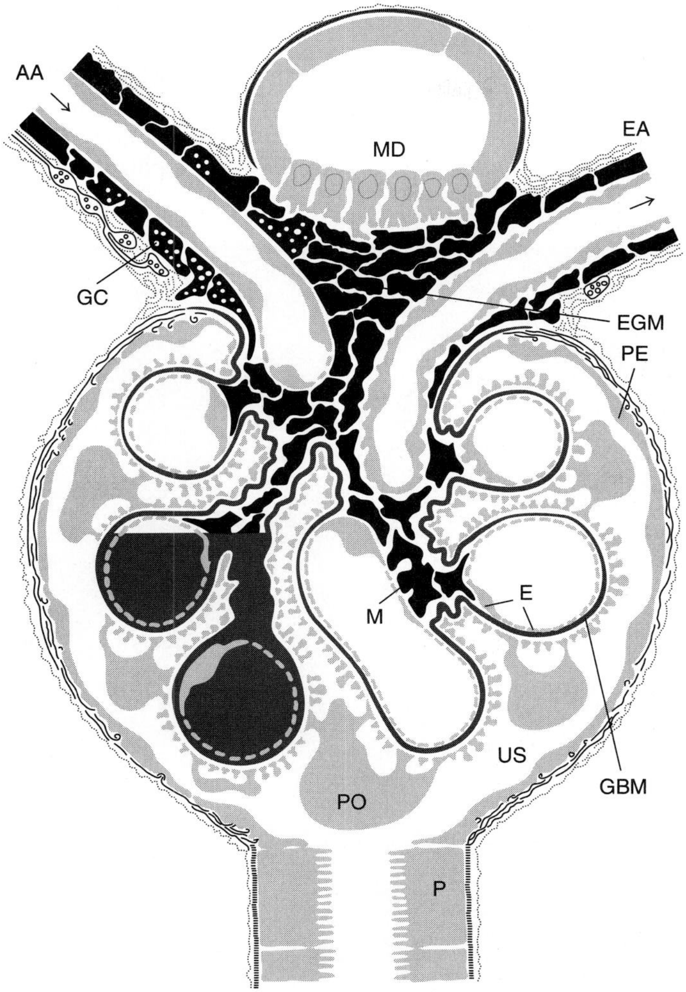

Figure 1–3. Diagram of a longitudinal section through a glomerulus and its juxtaglomerular (JG) apparatus. The JG apparatus consists of the granular cells (GC), which secrete renin, the macula densa (MD), and the extraglomerular mesangial cells (EGM). E, endothelium of the capillaries; EA, efferent arteriole; AA, afferent arteriole; PE, parietal (outer) epithelium of Bowman's space; PO, podocytes of Bowman's capsule; GBM, glomerular basement membrane. (Reproduced with permission from Kriz W et al. In: Davidson AM, ed. *Proceedings of the 10th International Congress on Nephrology, Vol 1.* London: Balliere Tindall; 1987.)

it is into this space that fluid filters. Opposite the vascular pole, Bowman's capsule has an opening that leads into the first portion of the tubule (see Figure 1–3, bottom).

The filtration barrier in the renal corpuscle through which all filtered substances must pass consists of 3 layers: the capillary endothelium of the glomerular capillaries, a rather thick basement membrane, and a single-celled layer of epithelial cells (Figure 1–4). The first layer, the endothelial cells of the capillaries, is perforated by

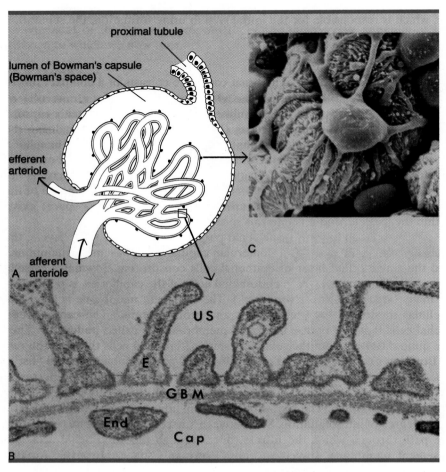

Figure 1–4. **A,** Anatomy of the glomerulus. **B,** Cross-section of glomerular membranes. US, "urinary" (Bowman's) space; E, epithelial foot processes; GBM, glomerular basement membranes; End, capillary endothelium; Cap, lumen of capillary. (Courtesy HG Rennke. Originally published in Fed Proc 1977;36:2019; reprinted with permission.) **C,** Scanning electron micrograph of podocytes covering glomerular capillary loops; the view is from inside Bowman's space. The large mass is a cell body. Note the remarkable interdigitation of the foot processes from adjacent podocytes and the slits between them. (Courtesy C Tisher.)

many large fenestrae ("windows"), like a slice of Swiss cheese, and is freely permeable to everything in the blood except red blood cells and platelets. The basement membrane in the middle is not a membrane in the sense of a lipid bilayer membrane but is a gel-like acellular meshwork of glycoproteins and proteoglycans, like a kitchen sponge. The epithelial cells that rest on the basement membrane and face Bowman's space are called *podocytes*. They are quite different from the relatively simple, flattened cells that line the outside of Bowman's capsule. The podocytes have an unusual octopus-like structure. Small "fingers," called *pedicels* (or foot processes), extend from each arm of the podocyte and are embedded in the basement membrane. Pedicels interdigitate with the pedicels from adjacent podocytes. Spaces between adjacent pedicels constitute the path through which the filtrate, once through the endothelial cells and basement membrane, travels to enter Bowman's space. The foot processes are coated by a thick layer of extracellular material, which partially occludes the slits, and extremely thin processes called *slit diaphragms* bridge the slits between the pedicels. These are like miniature ladders. The pedicels form the sides of the ladder, and the slit diaphragms are the rungs.

The functional significance of this anatomic arrangement is that it permits the filtration of large volumes of fluid from the capillaries into Bowman's space but restricts filtration of large plasma proteins such as albumin.

A third cell type—mesangial cells—is found in the central part of the glomerulus between and within capillary loops (see Figure 1–3). Glomerular mesangial cells act as phagocytes and remove trapped material from the basement membrane. They also contain large numbers of myofilaments and can contract in response to a variety of stimuli in a manner similar to vascular smooth muscle cells. The role of such contraction in influencing filtration by the renal corpuscles is discussed in Chapters 2 and 7.

The Tubule

Throughout its course, the *tubule* is made up of a single layer of epithelial cells resting on a basement membrane. (*Note:* All epithelial cell layers rest on a basement membrane). The structural and immunocytochemical characteristics of these epithelial cells vary from segment to segment of the tubule. A common feature is the presence of tight junctions between adjacent cells that physically link them together (like the plastic form that holds a six-pack of soft drinks together).

Table 1–1 lists the names and sequence of the various tubular segments, as illustrated in Figures 1–2 and 1–5. Physiologists and anatomists have traditionally grouped 2 or more contiguous tubular segments for purposes of reference, but the terminologies have varied considerably. Table 1–1 also gives the combination terms used in this text.

The *proximal tubule*, which drains Bowman's capsule, consists of a coiled segment—the proximal convoluted tubule—followed by a straight segment—the proximal straight tubule—which descends toward the medulla, perpendicular to the cortical surface of the kidney.

Table 1–1. Terminology for the tubular segments

Sequence of segments	Combination terms used in text
Proximal convoluted tubule Proximal straight tubule }	Proximal tubule
Descending thin limb of Henle's loop Ascending thin limb of Henle's loop Thick ascending limb of Henle's loop (contains macula densa near end) }	Henle's loop
Distal convoluted tubule	
Connecting tubule Cortical collecting duct Outer medullary collecting duct Inner medullary collecting duct (last portion is papillary duct) }	Collecting-duct system

The next segment, into which the proximal straight tubule drains, is the *descending thin limb of Henle's loop* (or simply the descending thin limb). The descending thin limb is in the medulla and is surrounded by an interstitial environment that is quite different from that in the cortex. The descending thin limb ends at a hairpin loop, and the tubule then begins to ascend parallel to the descending limb. The loops penetrate to varying depths within the medulla. In long loops (see later discussion), the epithelium of the first portion of this ascending limb remains thin, although different from that of the descending limb. This segment is called the *ascending thin limb of Henle's loop* (or simply the ascending thin limb) (see Figure 1–5). Beyond this segment, in these long loops, the epithelium thickens, and this next segment is called the *thick ascending limb of Henle's loop* (or simply the thick ascending limb). In short loops (see later discussion), there is no ascending thin limb, and the thick ascending limb begins right at the hairpin loop (see Figure 1–5). The thick ascending limb rises back into the cortex. Near the end of every thick ascending limb, the tubule returns to Bowman's capsule, from which it originated, and passes directly between the afferent and efferent arterioles, as they enter and exit that renal corpuscle at its vascular pole (see Figure 1–3). The cells in the thick ascending limb closest to Bowman's capsule (between the afferent and efferent arterioles) are specialized cells known as the *macula densa*. The macula densa marks the end of the thick ascending limb and the beginning of the distal convoluted tubule. This is followed by the connecting tubule, which leads to the cortical collecting tubule, the first portion of which is called the initial collecting tubule.

From Bowman's capsule through the loop of Henle to the initial collecting tubules, each of the 1 million nephrons in each kidney is completely separate from the others. However, connecting tubules from several nephrons merge to form cortical collecting tubules, and a number of initial collecting tubules then join end to end or side to side to form larger cortical collecting ducts. All the cortical collecting ducts then run downward to enter the medulla and become outer medullary collecting ducts and then inner medullary collecting ducts. The latter merge to form several hundred large

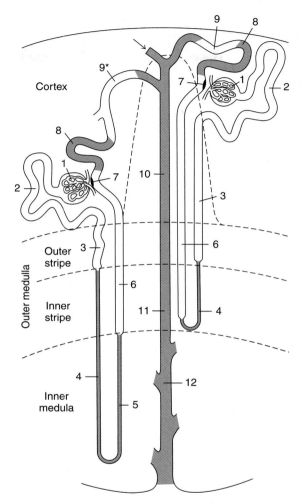

Figure 1–5. Standard nomenclature for structures of the kidney (1988 Commission of the International Union of Physiological Sciences). Shown are a short-looped and a long-looped (juxtamedullary) nephron, together with the collecting system (not drawn to scale). A cortical medullary ray—the part of the cortex that contains the straight proximal tubules, cortical thick ascending limbs, and cortical collecting ducts—is delineated by a dashed line. 1, renal corpuscle (Bowman's capsule and the glomerulus; 2, proximal convoluted tubule; 3, proximal straight tubule; 4, descending thin limb; 5, ascending thin limb; 6, thick ascending limb; 7, macula densa (located within the final portion of the thick ascending limb); 8, distal convoluted tubule; 9, connecting tubule; 9*, connecting tubule of a juxtamedullary nephron that arches upward to form a so-called arcade (there are only a few of these in the human kidney); 10, cortical collecting duct; 11, outer medullary collecting duct; 12, inner medullary collecting duct. (Reproduced with permission from Kriz W, Bankir L. Am J Physiol 1988;254LF:F1-F8.)

ducts, the last portions of which are called *papillary collecting ducts,* each of which empties into a calyx of the renal pelvis.

The pathway taken by fluids flowing within a nephron always begins in the cortex (in Bowman's capsule), descends into the medulla (descending limb of the loop of Henle), returns to the cortex (thick ascending limb of the loop of Henle), passes down into the medulla once more (medullary collecting tubule), and ends up in a renal calyx. Each renal calyx is continuous with the ureter, which empties into the urinary bladder, where urine is temporarily stored and from which it is intermittently eliminated. The urine is not altered after it enters a calyx. From this point on, the remainder of the urinary system serves only to maintain osmotic and solute gradients established by the kidney.

As noted earlier, the tubular epithelium has a one-cell thickness throughout. Before the distal convoluted tubule, the cells in any given segment are homogeneous and distinct for that segment. Thus, for example, the thick ascending limb contains only thick ascending limb cells. However, beginning in the second half of the distal convoluted tubule, 2 cell types are found in most of the remaining segments. One type constitutes the majority of cells in the particular segment, is considered specific for that segment, and is named accordingly: distal convoluted tubule cells, connecting tubule cells, and collecting-duct cells, the last known more commonly as *principal cells.* Interspersed among the segment-specific cells in each of these 3 segments are individual cells of the second type, called *intercalated cells.* To make things still more complicated, we will see that there are actually several types of intercalated cells; 2 of them are called type A and type B. (The last portion of the medullary collecting duct contains neither principal cells nor intercalated cells but is composed entirely of a distinct cell type called the *inner medullary collecting-duct cells.*)

Several simplifying conventions are used in this chapter and elsewhere in the textbook: (1) We will not usually distinguish between the convoluted and straight portions of the proximal tubule; (2) the functioning of the connecting tubule is generally similar to that of the cortical collecting tubule, and we tacitly lump them together as cortical collecting tubules.

BLOOD SUPPLY TO THE NEPHRONS

 Blood enters each kidney via a renal artery, which then divides into progressively smaller branches: interlobar, arcuate, and finally cortical radial arteries (also called interlobular arteries). As each of the cortical radial arteries projects toward the outer kidney surface, a series of parallel afferent arterioles branch off at right angles (Figure 1–6), each of which leads to a glomerulus. Note that these arteries and glomeruli are found only in the cortex, never in the medulla.

Normally only about 20% of the plasma (and none of the erythrocytes) entering the glomerulus is filtered from the glomerulus into Bowman's capsule. Where does the remaining blood go next? In almost all other organs, capillaries recombine to form the beginnings of the venous system, but the glomerular capillaries instead recombine to form another set of arterioles called the efferent arterioles. Thus, blood leaves each glomerulus through a single efferent arteriole at the vascular pole of Bowman's capsule (see Figure 1–3). The efferent arteriole soon subdivides into a second set of capillaries (see Figure 1–6). These are the peritubular capillaries, which are profusely distributed throughout the cortex. The peritubular capillaries then rejoin to form the veins by which blood ultimately leaves the kidney.

The vascular structures supplying the medulla differ from those in the cortex (see Figure 1–6). From many of the juxtamedullary glomeruli (the glomeruli lying just above the corticomedullary border), long efferent arterioles extend downward into the outer medulla, where they divide many times to form bundles of parallel vessels that penetrate deep into the medulla. These are called descending *vasa recta* (Latin *recta* for "straight" and *vasa* for "vessels"). Although it is still uncertain, a small fraction of the descending vasa recta may branch off from the cortical radial arteries before the glomeruli, not after. The vasa recta on the outside of the vascular bundles give rise to capillaries that surround Henle's loops and the collecting ducts in the outer medulla. The center-most vasa recta supply capillaries in the inner medulla. The capillaries from the inner medulla re-form into ascending vasa recta that run in close association with the descending vasa recta within the vascular bundles. The structural and functional properties of the vasa recta are rather complex. The beginnings of the descending vasa recta are like arterioles, containing smooth muscle in their walls, but become more capillary like as they descend. The ascending vasa recta have a fenestrated endothelium like that found in the glomerular capillaries. Therefore, the vasa recta, in addition to being conduits for blood, also participate in exchanging water and solutes between plasma and interstitium. The whole arrangement of descending and ascending blood flowing in parallel has major significance for the formation of concentrated urine (described in Chapter 6) because plasma constituents can exchange between descending and ascending vessels.

Categories of Nephrons

There are important regional differences in the various tubular segments of the nephron. All the renal corpuscles are in the cortex (accounting for its granular appearance) as well as the convoluted portions of the proximal tubule, cortical portions of Henle's loops, distal convoluted tubules, connecting tubules, and cortical collecting ducts. The medulla contains the medullary portions of Henle's loops and the medullary collecting ducts.

Nephrons are categorized according to the locations of their renal corpuscles in the cortex (see Figure 1–5): (1) In superficial cortical nephrons, renal corpuscles are located within 1 mm of the capsular surface of the kidneys; (2) in midcortical nephrons, renal corpuscles are located, as their name implies, in the midcortex, deep relative to the superficial cortical nephrons but above (3) the juxtamedullary nephrons, which, as mentioned previously, have renal corpuscles located just above the junction between cortex and medulla. One major distinction among these 3 categories of nephrons is the length of Henle's loop. All superficial cortical nephrons have short loops, which make their hairpin turn above the junction of outer and inner medulla. All juxtamedullary nephrons have long loops, which extend into the inner medulla, often to the tip of a papilla. Midcortical nephrons may be either short looped or long looped. The additional length

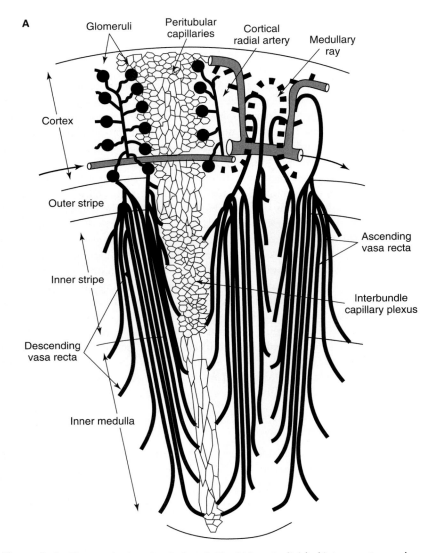

Figure 1–6. The renal microcirculation. **A,** The kidney is divided into a cortex and a medulla. The cortex contains an arterial network, glomeruli, a dense peritubular capillary plexus, and a venous drainage system. Not shown are Bowman's capsules surrounding the glomeruli, from which the proximal convoluted tubules exit at the urinary pole. The dashed line separates a medullary ray from the cortical labyrinth. An arcuate artery (arrow) gives rise to cortical radial (interlobular) arteries from which afferent arterioles originate at an angle that varies with cortical location. Blood is supplied to the peritubular capillaries of the cortex from the efferent flow out of superficial glomeruli. Blood is supplied to the medulla from the efferent flow out of juxtamedullary glomeruli. Efferent arterioles of juxtamedullary glomeruli give rise to descending vasa recta in the outer stripe of the outer medulla. In the inner stripe of the outer medulla, descending

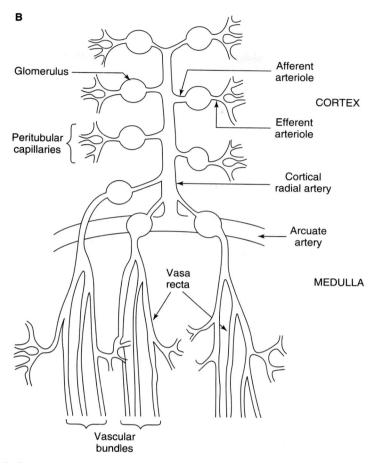

Figure 1-6. (Cont.) vasa recta and ascending vasa recta returning from the inner medulla form vascular bundles. The descending vasa recta from the bundle periphery supply the interbundle capillary plexus of the inner stripe, whereas those in the center supply blood to the capillaries of the inner medulla. **B,** Parts of the microcirculatory segments in the cortex and outer medulla are shown in greater detail.

of Henle's loop in long-looped nephrons is due to a longer descending thin limb and the presence of an ascending thin limb. Finally, the beginning of the thick ascending limb marks the border between the outer and inner medulla; in other words, the thick ascending limbs are found only in the cortex and outer medulla.

Nephron Heterogeneity

As stated earlier, there are more than 2 million nephrons in the 2 human kidneys. These nephrons manifest significant differences in anatomic, biochemical, and functional characteristics beyond those described in the previous section. For simplicity, however, we generally ignore these complexities, many of which currently are not fully understood.

The Juxtaglomerular Apparatus

Reference was made earlier to the macula densa, a portion of the late thick ascending limb at the point where, in all nephrons, this segment abuts the afferent and efferent arterioles at the vascular pole of the renal corpuscle from which the tubule arose. This entire area is known as the juxtaglomerular (JG) apparatus (see Figure 1–3). (Do not confuse the term *juxtaglomerular apparatus* with *juxtamedullary nephron.*) Each JG apparatus is made up of 3 cell types: (1) granular cells, which are differentiated smooth muscle cells in the walls of the afferent arterioles; (2) extraglomerular mesangial cells; and (3) macula densa cells, specialized thick ascending limb epithelial cells.

The granular cells (so called because they contain secretory vesicles that appear granular in light micrographs) are the cells that secrete the hormone renin, a crucial substance for control of renal function and blood pressure. The extraglomerular mesangial cells are morphologically similar to and continuous with the glomerular mesangial cells but lie outside Bowman's capsule. The macula densa cells are detectors of the luminal content of the nephron at the very end of the thick ascending limb and contribute to the control of glomerular filtration rate (GFR) and to the control of renin secretion.

Renal Innervation

The kidneys receive a rich supply of sympathetic neurons. These are distributed to the afferent and efferent arterioles, the JG apparatus, and many portions of the tubule. There is no significant parasympathetic innervation. There are some dopamine-containing neurons, the functions of which are uncertain.

BASIC RENAL PROCESSES

The working structures of the kidney are the nephrons and collecting tubules into which the nephrons drain. Figure 1–7 illustrates the meaning of several key words that we use to describe how the kidneys function. It is essential that any student of the kidney grasp their meaning.

Filtration is the process by which water and solutes in the blood leave the vascular system through the filtration barrier and enter Bowman's space (a space that is topologically outside the body). *Secretion* is the process of moving substances into the tubular lumen from the cytosol of epithelial cells that form the walls of the nephron. Secreted substances may originate by synthesis within the epithelial cells or, more often, by crossing the epithelial layer from the surrounding renal interstitium. *Reabsorption* is the process of moving substances from the lumen across the epithelial layer into the surrounding interstitium. In most cases, reabsorbed substances then move from the interstitium into surrounding blood vessels, so that the term *reabsorption* implies a two-step process of removal from the lumen

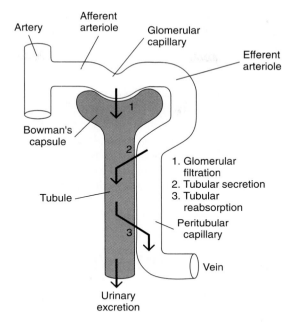

Figure 1–7. The 3 basic renal processes. Only the directions of reabsorption and secretion, not specific sites or order of occurrence, are shown. Depending on the specific substance, reabsorption and secretion can occur at various sites along the tubule.

followed by movement into the blood. *Excretion* means exit of the substance from the body (ie, the substance is present in the final urine produced by the kidneys). *Synthesis* means that a substance is constructed from molecular precursors, and *catabolism* means the substance is broken down into smaller component molecules.

The renal handling of any substance consists of some combination of the just-mentioned processes. If we can answer the following questions, we can know what the kidney does with a given substance. Is it filtered? Is it secreted? Is it reabsorbed? Is it synthesized? Is it catabolized?

Glomerular Filtration

Urine formation begins with glomerular filtration, the bulk flow of fluid from the glomerular capillaries into Bowman's capsule. The glomerular filtrate (ie, the fluid within Bowman's capsule) is very much like blood plasma. However, it contains very little total protein. The large plasma proteins like albumin and the globulins are virtually excluded from moving through the filtration barrier. Smaller proteins, such as many of the peptide hormones, are present in the filtrate, but their mass in total is miniscule compared with the mass of large plasma proteins in the blood. The filtrate contains most inorganic ions and low-molecular-weight organic solutes in virtually the same concentrations as in the plasma. Substances that are present in the filtrate at the same concentration as found in the plasma are said to be *freely filtered.*

Many low-molecular-weight components of blood are freely filtered. Among the most common substances included in the freely filtered category are the ions sodium, potassium, chloride, and bicarbonate; the neutral organics glucose and urea; amino acids; and peptides like insulin and antidiuretic hormone (ADH).

The volume of filtrate formed per unit time is known as the glomerular filtration rate (GFR). In a normal young adult male, the GFR is an incredible 180 L/day (125 mL/min)! Contrast this value with the net filtration of fluid across all the other capillaries in the body: approximately 4 L/day. The implications of this huge GFR are extremely important. When we recall that the average total volume of plasma in humans is approximately 3 L, it follows that the entire plasma volume is filtered by the kidneys some 60 times a day. The opportunity to filter such huge volumes of plasma enables the kidneys to excrete large quantities of waste products and to regulate the constituents of the internal environment very precisely.

The forces that determine the GFR and their physiological control are described in Chapters 2 and 7.

Tubular Reabsorption and Tubular Secretion

The volume and solute contents of the final urine that enters the renal pelvis are quite different from those of the glomerular filtrate. Clearly, almost all the filtered volume must be reabsorbed; otherwise, with a filtration rate of 180 L/day, we would urinate ourselves into dehydration very quickly. As the filtrate flows from Bowman's capsule through the various portions of the tubule, its composition is altered, mostly by removing material (tubular reabsorption) but also by adding material (tubular secretion). As described earlier, the tubule is, at all points, intimately associated with peritubular capillaries, a relationship that permits transfer of materials between the capillary plasma and the lumen of the tubule.

The most common relationships among these basic renal processes of glomerular filtration, tubular reabsorption, and tubular secretion are shown in the hypothetical examples of Figure 1–8. Plasma, containing 3 low-molecular-weight substances (X, Y, and Z), enters the glomerular capillaries, and approximately 20% of the plasma is filtered into Bowman's capsule. The filtrate contains substances X, Y, and Z in the same concentrations as the plasma (ie, each one is freely filtered). The filtrate enters the proximal convoluted tubule and begins its flow through the rest of the tubule. Simultaneously, the remaining 80% of the plasma, with its substances X, Y, and Z in the same concentrations as they had when entering the kidney, leaves the glomerular capillaries via the efferent arterioles and enters the peritubular capillaries.

Suppose the cells of the tubular epithelium can secrete all the peritubular-capillary substance X into the tubular lumen but cannot reabsorb substance X. Thus, by the combination of filtration and tubular secretion, all the plasma that originally entered the renal artery is cleared of substance X, which leaves the body via the urine. Now suppose the tubule can reabsorb some of substance Y. The amount of substance Y reabsorption is small, so most of the filtered substance Y escapes from the body in the urine. In contrast, let substance Z be reabsorbed fully. Therefore, no substance Z is lost from the body. Hence, the processes of filtration and reabsorption have canceled each other, and the net result is as though substance Z had never entered the kidney at all.

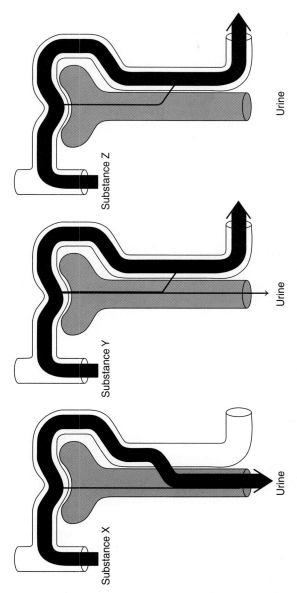

Figure 1–8. Renal manipulation of 3 hypothetical substances, X, Y, and Z. Substance X is filtered and secreted but not reabsorbed. Substance Z is filtered but is completely reabsorbed.

Table 1–2. Average values for several substances handled by filtration and reabsorption

Substance	Amount filtered per day	Amount excreted	% reabsorbed
Water, L	180	1.8	99.0
Sodium, g	630	3.2	99.5
Glucose, g	180	0	100
Urea, g	56	28	50

As we will see, most of the tubular transport consists of reabsorption rather than tubular secretion. An idea of the magnitude and importance of tubular reabsorption can be gained from Table 1–2, which summarizes data for a few plasma components that undergo reabsorption. The values in Table 1–2 are typical for a normal person on an average diet. There are at least 3 important generalizations to be drawn from this table:

1. Because of the huge GFR, the quantities filtered per day are enormous, generally larger than the amounts of the substances in the body. For example, the body contains about 40 L of water, but the volume of water filtered each day is 180 L. If reabsorption of water ceased but filtration continued, the total plasma water would be urinated within 30 min.

2. Reabsorption of waste products, such as urea, is incomplete, so that large fractions of their filtered amounts are excreted in the urine, like substance Y in our hypothetical example.

3. Reabsorption of most "useful" plasma components (eg, water, electrolytes, and glucose) varies from essentially complete, so that urine concentrations should normally be undetectable (eg, glucose), to almost complete (eg, water and most electrolytes), so that the amounts excreted in the urine represent only very small fractions of the filtered amounts.

For each plasma substance, a particular combination of filtration, reabsorption, and secretion applies. The relative proportions of these processes then determine the amount excreted. A critical point is that the rates at which the relevant processes proceed for many of these substances are subject to physiological control. By triggering changes in the rates of filtration, reabsorption, or secretion when the body content of a substance goes above or below normal, these mechanisms can regulate excretion to keep the body in balance. For example, consider what happens when a person drinks a large quantity of water: Within 1 to 2 h, all the excess water has been excreted in the urine, partly as the result of an increase in GFR but mainly as the result of decreased tubular reabsorption of water. The body is kept in balance for water by increasing excretion. By keeping the body in balance, the kidney is the effector organ of a reflex that maintains body water concentration within very narrow limits.

Metabolism by the Tubules

Although renal physiologists traditionally list glomerular filtration, tubular reabsorption, and tubular secretion as the 3 basic renal processes, we cannot overlook metabolism by the tubular cells. For example, the tubular cells may extract organic nutrients from the glomerular filtrate or peritubular capillaries and metabolize them as dictated by the cells' own nutrient requirements. In so doing, the renal cells are behaving no differently than any other cells in the body. In contrast, other metabolic transformations performed by the kidney are not directed toward its own nutritional requirements but rather toward altering the composition of the urine and plasma. The most important of these are the synthesis of ammonium from glutamine and the production of bicarbonate, both described in Chapter 9.

Regulation of Renal Function

By far, the most difficult aspect of renal physiology for students (and authors alike) is regulation of renal function. Neural signals, hormonal signals, and intrarenal chemical messengers combine to regulate the basic renal processes presented previously in a manner to help the kidneys meet the needs of the body. Unfortunately, our collective knowledge on much of this is, as yet, incomplete. Of necessity, much of the coverage in this textbook will attempt to draw an overview of renal function without an emphasis on nuance and detail that is more appropriate for advanced texts.

As with many organs, signals regulating the kidney arise from both neural and hormonal input. Neural signals originate in the sympathetic celiac plexus. Sympathetic signals exert major control over renal blood flow, glomerular filtration, and release of vasoactive substances (the renin-angiotensin system, described later). Hormonal signals originate in the adrenal gland, pituitary gland, and heart. The adrenal cortex secretes the steroid hormones aldosterone and cortisol, and the adrenal medulla secretes the catecholamines epinephrine and norepinephrine. All of these hormones, but mainly aldosterone, are regulators of sodium and potassium excretion by the kidney. The pituitary gland secretes the hormone arginine vasopressin (also called ADH). ADH is a major regulator of water excretion, and via its influence on the renal vasculature and possible collecting-duct principal cells, probably sodium excretion as well. The heart secretes hormones, natriuretic peptides, that contribute to signaling increased excretion of sodium by the kidneys. The most difficult aspect of regulation lies in the realm of *intrarenal* chemical messengers (ie, messengers that originate in one part of the kidney and act in another part). It is clear that an array of substances (eg, nitric oxide, purinergic agonists, various eicosanoids) influence basic renal processes, but, for the most part, the role of these substances is beyond the scope of this text.

Overview of Regional Function

We conclude this chapter with a broad overview of the tasks performed by the various nephron segments. Later, we examine renal function substance by substance and see how tasks performed in the various regions combine to produce an overall result that is useful for the body.

The glomerulus is the site of filtration—about 180 L/day of volume and proportional amounts of solutes that are freely filtered, which is the case for most solutes (large plasma proteins are an exception). The glomerulus is where the greatest mass of excreted substances enter the nephron. The proximal tubule (convoluted and straight portions) reabsorbs about two thirds of the filtered water, sodium, and chloride. The proximal convoluted tubule reabsorbs all of the useful organic molecules that the body wishes to conserve (eg, glucose, amino acids). It reabsorbs significant fractions, but by no means all, of many important ions, such as potassium, phosphate, calcium, and bicarbonate. It is the site of secretion of a number of organic substances that are either metabolic waste products (eg, urate, creatinine) or drugs (eg, penicillin) that physicians must replace to make up for renal excretion.

The loop of Henle contains different segments that perform different functions, but the key functions occur in the thick ascending limb (a region that begins in the outer medulla for all nephrons and continues outward into the renal cortex until it reaches the renal corpuscle from which the tubule arose (which can, depending on the nephron, be near the corticomedullary border or close to the cortical surface)). As a whole, the loop of Henle reabsorbs about 20% of the filtered sodium and chloride and 10% of the filtered water. A crucial consequence of these different proportions is that, by reabsorbing relatively more salt than water, the luminal fluid becomes *diluted* relative to normal plasma and the surrounding interstitium. During periods when the kidneys excrete dilute final urine, the role of the loop of Henle in diluting the luminal fluid is crucial.

The end of the loop of Henle contains cells of the macula densa, which senses or assays the sodium and chloride content of the lumen and generates signals that influence other aspects of renal function, specifically the renin-angiotensin system (discussed in Chapter 7).

The distal tubule and connecting tubule together reabsorb some additional salt and water, perhaps 5% of each.

The cortical collecting tubule is where several (6–10) connecting tubules join to form 1 tubule. Cells of the cortical collecting tubule are strongly responsive to and are regulated by the hormones aldosterone and ADH. Aldosterone enhances sodium reabsorption and potassium secretion by this segment, and ADH enhances water reabsorption. The degree to which these processes are stimulated or not stimulated plays a major role in regulating the amount of solutes and water present in the final urine. With large amounts of ADH present, most of the water remaining in the lumen is reabsorbed, leading to concentrated, low-volume urine. With little ADH present, most of the water passes on to the final urine, producing dilute, high-volume urine.

The medullary collecting tubule continues the functions of the cortical collecting tubule in salt and water reabsorption. In addition, it plays a major role in regulating urea reabsorption and in acid-base balance (secretion of protons or bicarbonate).

KEY CONCEPTS

One major function of the kidneys is to regulate excretion of substances at a rate that exactly balances their input into the body and, thereby, maintain total body homeostatic balance for many substances.

A second major function of the kidneys is to regulate blood volume, blood osmolarity, and total body sodium content in a way that determines average blood pressure.

The working tissues of the kidney are divided into an outer cortex and inner medulla.

Each functional renal unit is composed of a filtering component (glomerulus) and a transporting tubular component (the nephron and collecting duct).

The cortex receives an enormous volume of blood that flows in series through glomerular capillaries and then peritubular capillaries, whereas blood flow to the medulla is highly restricted.

The renal handling of any substance is defined by its rate of filtration, reabsorption, secretion, and, in some cases, metabolism.

STUDY QUESTIONS

1–1. Is the following statement true or false? The difference between superficial and juxtamedullary nephrons is that the former have their glomeruli in the cortex whereas the glomeruli of the latter are in the medulla.

1–2. What percentage of the blood entering the kidney flows directly into the medulla without passing through the cortex?

1–3. Substance T is present in the urine. Does this prove that it entered the renal tubule by filtration at the glomerulus?

1–4. Substance V is not normally present in the urine. Does this prove that it is neither filtered nor secreted?

1–5. A substance is filtered into Bowman's space and excreted in the urine. How many cell plasma membranes must it cross in order to exit the body?

1–6. A substance is freely filtered. Does this mean that it is all filtered?

1–7. If you immunologically labeled cells of the macula densa, would you find the label in the cortex, medulla, or both?

1–8. Given the generalizations about transport events in the medulla (secretion, reabsorption), can you say that blood flow into the medulla is in any way different in volume than blood flow out of the medulla?

Renal Blood Flow and Glomerular Filtration

OBJECTIVES

The student understands the hemodynamics of renal blood flow.

▶ Defines renal blood flow, renal plasma flow, glomerular filtration rate, and filtration fraction, and gives normal values.

▶ States the formula relating flow, pressure, and resistance in an organ.

▶ Describes the relative resistances of the afferent arterioles and efferent arterioles.

▶ Describes the effects of changes in afferent and efferent arteriolar resistances on renal blood flow.

The student understands how glomerular filtrate is formed and the forces that determine its rate of formation.

▶ Describes how molecular size and electrical charge determine filterability of plasma solutes; states how protein binding of a low-molecular-weight substance influences its filterability.

▶ States the formula for the determinants of glomerular filtration rate, and states, in qualitative terms why the net filtration pressure is positive.

▶ Defines filtration coefficient and states how mesangial cells might alter the filtration coefficient; states the reason glomerular filtration rate is so large relative to filtration across other capillaries in the body.

▶ Describes how arterial pressure, afferent arteriolar resistance, and efferent arteriolar resistance influence glomerular capillary pressure.

▶ Describes how changes in renal plasma flow influence average glomerular capillary oncotic pressure.

The student understands the normal controls of renal blood flow and glomerular filtration rate.

▶ States the Starling forces involved in capillary filtration.

▶ States how changes in each Starling force affect glomerular filtration rate.

▶ Defines autoregulation of renal blood flow and glomerular filtration rate.

▶ Describes the myogenic and tubuloglomerular feedback mechanisms of autoregulation.

GLOMERULAR FILTRATION AND RENAL BLOOD FLOW

The kidneys receive an enormous blood flow: more than 1 L/min, or about 20% of the cardiac output. This blood flow is far in excess of the kidney's metabolic need and provides the kidneys with the flexibility to alter blood flow in response to physiological demand. All of this blood flows through glomeruli in the cortex.[1] The vast majority continues on (via efferent arterioles) to peritubular capillaries in the cortex and then into the renal venous system. A much smaller fraction, about 5–10%, flows from efferent arterioles down into the medulla. This medullary blood derives from juxtamedullary glomeruli that are situated near the corticomedullary border. Let us look at some typical numbers. A normal hematocrit is 0.45, and a typical renal blood flow (RBF) is 1.1 L/min. The renal plasma flow (RPF) = 0.55 × 1.1 L/min = 605 mL/min. As stated in Chapter 1, a typical glomerular filtration rate (GFR) is about 125 mL/min. Thus, of the 605 mL of plasma that enters the glomeruli via the afferent arterioles, 125/605, or 20%, filters into Bowman's space. The remaining 480 mL passes via the efferent arterioles into the peritubular capillaries. This ratio—GFR/RPF—is known as the *filtration fraction*. Because freely filtered substances are passing into Bowman's space along with the water, about 20% of all freely filtered substances (eg, sodium) that enter the kidney also move into Bowman's space.

FLOW, RESISTANCE, AND PRESSURE IN THE KIDNEYS

The basic equation for blood flow through any organ is as follows:

$$Q = \Delta P / R,$$

where Q is organ blood flow, ΔP is mean pressure in the artery supplying the organ minus mean pressure in the vein draining that organ, and R is the total vascular resistance in that organ. Resistance is determined by the blood viscosity and the lengths and radii of the organ's blood vessels, the arteriolar radii being overwhelmingly the major contributor. As described by Poiseiulle's law, resistance of a cylindrical vessel varies inversely with the fourth power of vessel radius. It takes only a 19% decrease or increase in vessel radius to double or halve vessel resistance. The radii of arterioles are regulated by the state of contraction of the arteriolar smooth muscle.

The presence of 2 sets of arterioles (afferent and efferent) and 2 sets of capillaries (glomerular and peritubular) makes the vasculature of the cortex unusual. (The vasculature of the medulla is even more unusual, but we concentrate on the cortex for now.) Normally, the resistances of the afferent and efferent arterioles are approximately equal and account for most of the total renal vascular resistance. Resistance in arteries preceding afferent arterioles (ie, cortical radial arteries) plays some role also, but we concentrate on the arterioles. Vascular pressures (ie, hydrostatic or hydraulic pressure) in the 2 capillary beds are quite different. The peritubular capillaries are downstream from the efferent arteriole and have a lower

---

[1] There is some evidence that a small fraction of blood approaching Bowman's capsule in afferent arterioles is diverted directly to the medulla without going through glomeruli. This fraction, if it exists at all, is small.

hydraulic pressure. Typical glomerular pressures are near 60 mm Hg in a normal unstressed individual, whereas peritubular pressures are closer to 20 mm Hg. The high glomerular pressure is crucial for glomerular filtration, whereas the low peritubular capillary pressure is equally crucial for the tubular reabsorption of fluid.

To repeat, total RBF is determined mainly by the mean pressure in the renal artery and the contractile state of the smooth muscle of the renal arterioles of the cortex. Now for a simple but very important point: A change in arteriolar resistance produces the same effect on RBF regardless of whether it occurs in the afferent arteriole or efferent arteriole. Because these vessels are in series, a change in either one has the same effect on the total. When the 2 resistances both change in the same direction, the most common state of affairs, their effects on RBF will be additive. When they change in different directions—one resistance increasing and the other decreasing—they exert opposing effects on RBF. We see in the next section that the story is totally different for GFR.

GLOMERULAR FILTRATION

Formation of Glomerular Filtrate

As stated in Chapter 1, the glomerular filtrate is nearly protein free[2] and contains most inorganic ions and low-molecular-weight organic solutes in virtually the same concentrations as in the plasma.

The filtration barrier within the glomerulus is the interface between the blood and the external world. The route that a filtered substances takes from the blood through the filtration barrier of a renal corpuscle into Bowman's space is a 3-step process: through fenestrae in the glomerular-capillary endothelial layer, through the basement membrane, and finally through slit diaphragms between podocyte foot processes. The portion of endothelial surface area occupied by fenestrae is about 10%. Just which of these structures constitute the major barriers to filtration of macromolecules has proven a difficult question to answer, but it is clear that they do so on the basis of both *molecular size* and *electrical charge*. Let us look first at size.

The filtration barrier of the renal corpuscle provides no hindrance to the movement of molecules with molecular weights less than 7000 d (ie, solutes this small are all freely filtered). This includes all small ions, glucose, urea, amino acids, and many hormones. The filtration barrier almost totally excludes plasma albumin (molecular weight of approximately 66,000 d). (We are, for simplicity, using molecular weight as our reference for size; in reality, it is molecular radius that is critical.) The hindrance to plasma albumin is not 100%, however, and so the glomerular filtrate does contain extremely small quantities of albumin, on the order of 10 mg/L or less. This is only about 0.02% of the concentration of albumin in plasma and is the reason for the use of the phrase "nearly protein-free" earlier. (*Note:* Some small substances are partly or mostly bound to large plasma proteins and are thus not free to be filtered, even though, when not bound to plasma proteins, they can easily move through the

---

[2] It is protein free in the sense that the total concentration of protein is very low. However, many small proteins that have low plasma concentrations, such as many peptide hormones, are freely or nearly freely filtered.

filtration barrier. This includes hydrophobic hormones of the steroid and thyroid categories and about 40% of the calcium in the blood.)

For molecules with a molecular weight ranging from 7000 and 70,000 d, the amount filtered becomes progressively smaller as the molecule becomes larger. Thus, many normally occurring plasma peptides and small proteins are filtered to a significant degree. Moreover, when certain small proteins not normally present in the plasma appear because of disease (eg, hemoglobin released from damaged erythrocytes or myoglobin released from damaged muscles), considerable filtration of these may occur.

Electrical charge is the second variable determining filterability of macromolecules. For any given size, negatively charged macromolecules are filtered to a lesser extent, and positively charged macromolecules to a greater extent, than neutral molecules. This is because the surfaces of all the components of the filtration barrier (the cell coats of the endothelium, the basement membrane, and the cell coats of the podocytes) contain fixed polyanions, which repel negatively charged macromolecules during filtration. Because almost all plasma proteins bear net negative charges, this electrical repulsion plays a very important restrictive role, enhancing that of purely size hindrance. (For example, when neutral dextrans the same size as plasma albumin are administered to experimental animals, they are found to be 5–10% filterable rather than albumin's 0.02%.) In other words, if albumin were not charged or the filtration barrier were not charged, even albumin would be filtered to a considerable degree. Certain diseases that cause glomerular capillaries to become "leaky" to protein do so by eliminating negative charges in the membranes.

It must be emphasized that the negative charges in the filtration membranes act as a hindrance only to macromolecules, not to mineral ions or low-molecular-weight organic solutes. Thus, chloride and bicarbonate ions, despite their negative charge, are freely filtered.

Direct Determinants of GFR

Variation in GFR is a crucial determinant of renal function.

 Everything else being equal, a higher GFR means greater excretion of salt and water. Regulation of the GFR is straightforward in terms of physical principles but very complex functionally because there are so many regulated variables. The rate of filtration in any of the body's capillaries, including the glomeruli, is determined by the hydraulic permeability of the capillaries, their surface area, and the net filtration pressure (NFP) acting across them.

$$\text{Rate of filtration} = \text{hydraulic permeability} \times \text{surface area} \times \text{NFP}$$

Because it is difficult to estimate the area of a capillary bed, a parameter called the filtration coefficient (K_f) is used to denote the product of the hydraulic permeability and the area.

The net filtration pressure is the algebraic sum of the hydrostatic pressures and the osmotic pressures resulting from protein—the oncotic, or colloid osmotic pressures (for additional description of the importance of oncotic

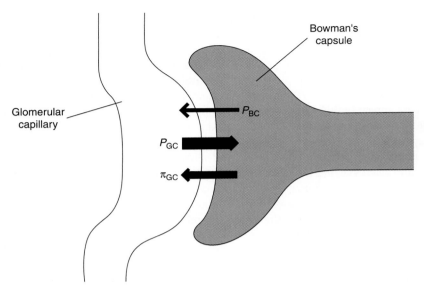

Figure 2–1. Net filtration pressure in the renal corpuscle equals glomerular-capillary hydraulic pressure (P_{GC}) minus Bowman's capsule hydraulic pressure (P_{BC}) minus glomerular-capillary oncotic pressure (π_{GC}).

pressure, see Chapter 4)–on the 2 sides of the capillary wall. There are 4 pressures to contend with: 2 hydrostatic pressures and 2 oncotic pressures. These are referred to as *Starling forces,* named after the physiologist who first described them. Applying this to the glomerular capillaries:

$$NFP = (P_{GC} - \pi_{GC}) - (P_{BC} - \pi_{BC})$$

where P_{GC} is glomerular capillary hydraulic pressure, π_{BC} is oncotic pressure of fluid in Bowman's capsule, P_{BC} is hydraulic pressure in Bowman's capsule, and π_{GC} is oncotic pressure in glomerular capillary plasma, shown schematically in Figure 2–1.

Because there is normally little protein in Bowman's capsule, π_{BC} may be taken as zero and not considered in our analysis. Accordingly, the overall equation for GFR becomes

$$GFR = K_f \cdot (P_{GC} - P_{BC} - \pi_{GC}).$$

The hydrostatic pressures in glomerular capillaries and Bowman's capsule have not been directly measured in humans. However, several lines of indirect evidence suggest that the human values are probably similar to those for the dog, and these values are shown in Table 2–1 and Figure 2–2 along with glomerular capillary oncotic pressure.

Note that the hydraulic pressure changes only slightly along the glomeruli; this is because the very large total cross-sectional area of the glomeruli collectively provides only a small resistance to flow. Importantly, note that the oncotic pressure in

Table 2–1. Estimated forces involved in glomerular filtration in humans

Forces	Afferent end of glomerular capillary (mm Hg)	Efferent end of glomerular capillary (mm Hg)
1 Favoring filtration Glomerular-capillary hydraulic pressure, P_{GC}	60	58
2 Opposing filtration a Hydraulic pressure in Bowman's capsule, P_{BC}	15	15
b Oncotic pressure in glomerular capillary, π_{GC}	21	33
3 Net filtration pressure (1 − 2)	24	10

the glomerular capillaries does change substantially along the length of the glomeruli. Water is moving out of the vascular space and leaving protein behind, thereby raising protein concentration and, hence, the oncotic pressure of the unfiltered plasma remaining in the glomerular capillaries. Mainly because of this large increase in oncotic pressure, the net filtration pressure decreases from the beginning of the glomerular capillaries to the end. The average net filtration pressure over the whole

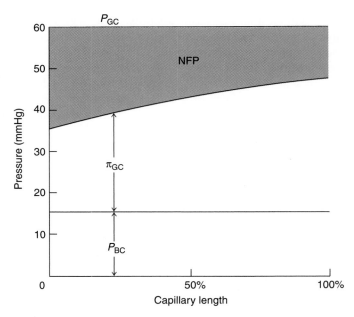

Figure 2–2. Estimated forces involved in glomerular filtration in humans (these are the same values shown Table 2–1). Net filtration pressure (NFP) $= P_{GC} - \pi_{GC} - P_{BC}$.

Table 2–2. Summary of direct GFR determinants and factors that influence them

Direct determinants of GFR: $GFR = K_f(P_{GC} - P_{BC} - \pi_{GC})$			Major factors that tend to increase the magnitude of the direct determinant
K_f	1.	↑	Glomerular surface area (because of relaxation of glomerular mesangial cells) Result: ↑ GFR
P_{GC}	1.	↑	Renal arterial pressure
	2.	↓	Afferent-arteriolar resistance (afferent dilation)
	3.	↑	Efferent-arteriolar resistance (efferent constriction) Result: ↑ GFR
P_{BC}	1.	↑	Intratubular pressure because of obstruction of tubule or extrarenal urinary system Result: ↓ GFR
π_{GC}	1.	↑	Systemic-plasma oncotic pressure (sets π_{GC} at beginning of glomerular capillaries)
	2.	↓	Renal plasma flow (causes increased rise of π_{GC} along glomerular capillaries) Result: ↓ GFR

GFR, glomerular filtration rate; K_f, filtration coefficient; P_{GC}, glomerular-capillary hydraulic pressure; P_{BC}, Bowman's capsule hydraulic pressure; π_{GC}, glomerular-capillary oncotic pressure. A reversal of all arrows in the table will cause a decrease in the magnitudes of K_f, P_{GC}, P_{BC}, and π_{GC}.

length of the glomerulus is about 17 mm Hg. This average net filtration pressure is higher than found in most nonrenal capillary beds. Along with a high value for K_f, it accounts for the enormous filtration of 180 L of fluid/day (compared with 3 L/day or so in all other capillary beds combined.)

As we have noted, the GFR is not fixed but shows marked fluctuations in differing physiological states and in disease. If all other factors remain constant, any change in K_f, P_{GC}, P_{BC}, or π_{GC} will alter GFR. However, "all other factors" do not always remain constant, and so other simultaneous events may oppose the effect of any one factor. To grasp this situation, it is essential to see how a change in any one factor affects GFR under the assumption that all other factors are held constant.

Table 2–2 presents a summary of these factors. It provides, in essence, a checklist to review when trying to understand how diseases or vasoactive chemical messengers and drugs change GFR. In this regard, it should be noted that the major cause of decreased GFR in renal disease is not any change in these parameters within individual nephrons but rather simply a decrease in the number of functioning nephrons.

K_f

Changes in K_f can be caused by glomerular disease and drugs, but this variable is also subject to normal physiological control by a variety of chemical messengers. The details are still not completely clear, but these messengers cause contraction of glomerular mesangial cells. Such contraction may restrict flow through some of the capillary loops, effectively reducing the area available for filtration and, hence, K_f. This decrease in K_f will tend to lower GFR.

P_{GC}

Hydrostatic pressure in the glomerular capillaries (P_{GC}) is the most complex of the variables in the basic filtration equation because it is itself influenced by so many factors. We can help depict the situation by using the analogy of a leaking garden hose. If pressure feeding the hose (pressure in the pipes leading to the faucet) goes up or down, this directly affects pressure in the hose and, hence, the rate of leak. Resistances in the hose also affect the leak. If we kink the hose upstream from the leak, pressure at the region of leak falls and less water leaks out. However, if we kink the hose beyond the leak, this *raises* pressure at the region of leak and increases leak rate. These same principles apply to P_{GC} and GFR. First, a change in renal arterial pressure will cause a change in P_{GC} in the same direction. If resistances remain constant, P_{GC} will rise and fall as renal artery pressure rises and falls. This is a crucial point because a major regulator of renal function is arterial blood pressure. Second, changes in the resistance of the afferent and efferent arterioles have *opposite* effects on P_{GC}. An increase in resistance *upstream* from the glomerulus in the afferent arteriole (like kinking the hose above the leak) will lower P_{GC}, whereas an increase in resistance *downstream* from the glomerulus in the efferent arteriole (like kinking the hose beyond the leak) will increase P_{GC}. In contrast, a decrease in afferent resistance (R_A) (resulting from afferent arteriolar dilation) will tend to raise P_{GC}. Similarly, a decrease in efferent resistance (R_E) (caused by efferent arteriolar dilation) tends to lower P_{GC}. It should also be clear that when R_A and R_E both change simultaneously in the same direction (ie, both increase or decrease), they exert opposing effects on P_{GC}.

It is possible for both resistances to rise by the same fraction, with the result that there is no effect on P_{GC} (even though, in this case, RBF would fall). In contrast, when they change in different directions, they cause additive effects on P_{GC} (and can have no effect on RBF). The real significance for this is that the kidney can regulate P_{GC} and, hence, GFR independently of RBF. The effect of changes in R_A and R_E are summarized in Figure 2–3.

P_{BC}

Changes in this variable generally are of very minor physiological importance. The major pathological cause of increased hydraulic pressure in Bowman's capsule is obstruction anywhere along the tubule or in the external portions of the urinary system (eg, the ureter). The effect of such an occlusion is to increase the tubular pressure everywhere proximal to the occlusion, all the way back to Bowman's capsule. The result is to decrease GFR.

π_{GC}

Oncotic pressure in the plasma at the very beginning of the glomerular capillaries is, of course, simply the oncotic pressure of systemic arterial plasma. Accordingly, a decrease in arterial plasma protein concentration, as occurs, for example, in liver disease, will lower arterial oncotic pressure and tend to increase GFR, whereas increased arterial oncotic pressure will tend to reduce GFR.

However, now recall that π_{GC} is identical to arterial oncotic pressure only at the very beginning of the glomerular capillaries; π_{GC} then progressively increases along the glomerular capillaries as protein-free fluid filters out of the capillary, concentrating

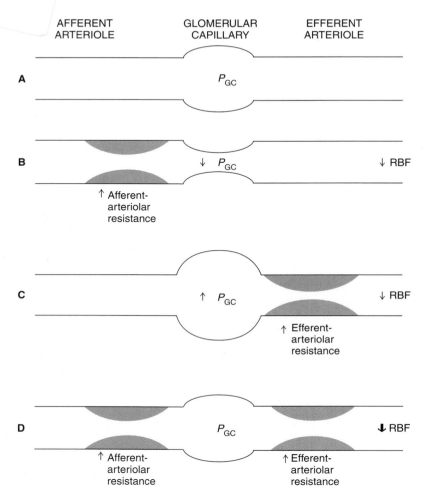

AFFERENT
ARTERIOLE

GLOMERULAR
CAPILLARY

EFFERENT
ARTERIOLE

A P_{GC}

B ↓ P_{GC} ↓ RBF

↑ Afferent-
arteriolar
resistance

C ↑ P_{GC} ↓ RBF

↑ Efferent-
arteriolar
resistance

D P_{GC} ↓ RBF

↑ Afferent-
arteriolar
resistance

↑ Efferent-
arteriolar
resistance

Figure 2–3. Effects of afferent- and/or efferent-arteriolar constriction on glomerular capillary pressure (P_{GC}) and renal blood flow (RBF). The RBF changes reflect changes in *total* renal arteriolar resistance, the location of the change being irrelevant. In contrast, the changes in P_{GC} are reflected in which set of arterioles the altered resistance occurs. Pure afferent constriction lowers both P_{GC} and RBF, whereas pure efferent constriction raises P_{GC} and lowers RBF. Simultaneous constriction of both afferent and efferent arterioles has counteracting effects on P_{GC} but additive effects on RBF; the effect on P_{GC} may be a small increase, small decrease, or no change. Vasodilation of only 1 set of arterioles would have effects on P_{GC} and RBF opposite those shown in parts B and C. Vasodilation of both sets would cause little or no change in P_{GC}, the same result as constriction of both sets but would cause a large increase in RBF. Constriction of 1 set of arterioles and dilation of the other would have maximal effects on P_{GC} but little effect on RBF.

the protein left behind. This means that net filtration pressure and, hence, filtration progressively decrease along the capillary length. Accordingly, anything that causes a steeper rise in π_{GC} will tend to lower average net filtration pressure and hence GFR.

This steep increase in oncotic pressure tends to occur when RPF is low. It should not be hard to visualize that the filtration of a given volume of fluid from a small total volume of plasma flowing through the glomeruli will cause the protein left behind to become more concentrated than if the total volume of plasma were large. In other words, a low RPF, all other factors remaining constant, will cause the π_{GC} to rise more steeply and reach a final value at the end of the glomerular capillaries, which is higher than normal. This increase in average π_{GC} along the capillaries lowers average net filtration pressure and, hence, GFR. Conversely, a high RPF, all other factors remaining constant, will cause π_{GC} to rise less steeply and reach a final value at the end of the capillaries that is less than normal, which will increase the GFR.

Another way of thinking about this is in terms of filtration fraction: the ratio GFR/RPF. The increase in π_{GC} along the glomerular capillaries is directly proportional to the filtration fraction (ie, the more volume that is filtered from plasma, the higher is the rise in π_{GC}. Therefore, if you know that filtration fraction has changed, you can be certain that there has also been a proportional change in π_{GC} and that this has played a role in altering GFR.

FILTERED LOAD

A term we use in other chapters is *filtered load*. It is the amount of substance that is filtered per unit time. For freely filtered substances, the filtered load is just the product of GFR and plasma concentration. Consider sodium. Its normal plasma concentration is 140 mEq/L, or 0.14 mEq/mL. (*Note:* 1 mEq of sodium is 1 mmol.) A normal GFR is 125 mL/min, so the filtered load of sodium is 0.14 mEq/mL × 125 mL/min = 17.5 mEq/min. We can do the same calculation for any other substance, being careful in each case to be aware of the unit of measure in which concentration is expressed. The filtered load is what is presented to the rest of the nephron to handle. A high filtered load means a substantial amount of material to be reabsorbed. The filtered load varies with plasma concentration and GFR. A rise in GFR, at constant plasma concentration, increases the filtered load, as does a rise in plasma concentration at constant GFR.

AUTOREGULATION

It is extremely important for the kidneys to keep the GFR at a level appropriate for the body because, as we have emphasized, the excretion of salt and water is strongly influenced by the GFR. We have also emphasized that the GFR is strongly influenced by renal arterial pressure. A rise in blood pressure causes an increased excretion of salt and water, a process called *pressure natriuresis* (see Chapter 7), whereas a fall in blood pressure diminishes excretion. These changes in excretion are mediated partly via changes in GFR. The effect is so strong that urinary excretion would tend to vary widely with the ordinary daily excursions of arterial pressure.

 However, changes in GFR and RBF are severely blunted by mechanisms that we collectively call *autoregulation*. Consider first a situation in which mean arterial pressure rises 20%. Such a modest rise occurs many times throughout the day in association with changes in excitement level and activity. Pretend, for the moment, that all renal vascular resistances remain constant. By the basic flow equation ($Q = \Delta P/R$), RBF would rise 20% also (actually slightly more if pressure in the renal vein is unaffected). What would this do to GFR? It would rise much more than 20%, in fact almost 50%. This is because net filtration pressure would rise almost 50%. In effect, fractional changes in upstream pressure (in the renal artery) are *magnified* in terms of net filtration pressure. Why is this? At the beginning of the glomerulus, capillary hydrostatic pressure is about 60 mm Hg, and net filtration pressure is about 24 mm Hg. With an increase in arterial pressure to 120 mm Hg, capillary pressure would rise to about 71 mm Hg, but there would be no increase in the pressures that oppose filtration—plasma oncotic pressure and Bowman's capsule pressure. Therefore, net filtration pressure would rise to about 35 mm Hg (an increase of almost 50%). The higher net filtration pressure would cause a parallel increase in GFR. (In turn, this would raise plasma oncotic pressure at the *distal* end of the glomerulus, tending to reduce filtration somewhat, but the total effect is still a major rise in GFR.) This emphasizes the crucial role of glomerular capillary pressure in glomerular filtration.

Now, what actually happens in the face of changes in mean arterial pressure? As is the case in many organs, blood flow does not change in proportion to changes in arterial pressure. The changes are blunted. A rise in driving pressure is counteracted by a rise in vascular resistance that *almost* offsets the rise in pressure. The word "almost" is crucial here. Higher driving pressures lead to higher flow but not proportionally. Consider Figure 2–4. Within the range of mean arterial pressures commonly found in the human body (between the dashed vertical lines in Figure 2–4),

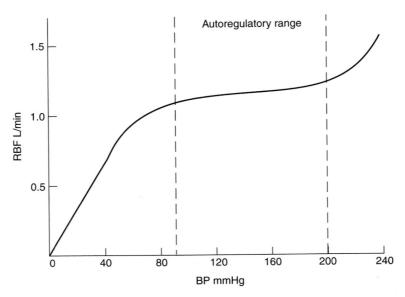

Figure 2–4. Autoregulation of renal blood flow (RBF). A similar pattern holds for glomerular filtration rate.

RBF varies only modestly when mean arterial pressure changes. This is partly a result of a direct reaction of the vascular smooth muscle to stretch or relaxation—or the *myogenic* response—and partly the result of intrarenal signals that we describe shortly. In addition to keeping changes in RBF fairly small, autoregulatory processes also keep changes in GFR fairly small. Again, GFR *does* rise with an increase in arterial pressure, just not substantially.

How do the intrarenal processes work? Much is by way of a process with the clumsy name of *tubuloglomerular feedback*. Tubuloglomerular feedback is feedback from the tubules back to the glomerulus (ie, an influence of events in the tubules on events in the glomeruli). We return to the mechanism in Chapter 7, but for now the essence of tubuloglomerular feedback can be summarized as follows: As the filtration rate in an individual nephron increases or decreases, the amount of sodium that escapes reabsorption in the proximal tubule and loop of Henle also increases or decreases. More sodium filtered means more sodium remaining in the lumen of the nephron and more sodium flowing from the thick ascending limb into the distal tubule. Recall that at the division between these nephron segments lies the macula densa, a special group of cells in the nephron wall where the nephron passes between the afferent and efferent arterioles (see Figure 1–7). The macula densa cells sense the amount of sodium and chloride in the lumen. They act, in part, as salt detectors. One result of changing levels of luminal sodium chloride is to increase or decrease the secretion of transmitter agents into the interstitial space that affect the filtration in the nearby glomerulus. High levels of sodium flowing past the macula densa cause a decrease in filtration rate; low levels of sodium flowing past allow a higher filtration rate. It is as though each nephron adjusts its filtration so that the right amount of sodium remains in the lumen to flow past the macula densa. How can it adjust its filtration? The transmitter agents released by the salt-sensing macula densa cells produce vasoconstriction of the afferent arteriole, thereby reducing hydrostatic pressure in the glomerular capillaries. These same agents also produce contraction of glomerular mesangial cells, thereby reducing the effective filtration coefficient. Both processes reduce the single-nephron filtration rate and keep it at a level appropriate for the rest of the nephron.

In conclusion, we emphasize that autoregulation blunts or lowers the RBF and GFR responses to changes in arterial pressure but does not totally prevent those changes.

KEY CONCEPTS

1. RBF is much higher than required for metabolic needs and is regulated for functional reasons, not metabolic demand.

2. RBF varies with driving pressure and varies inversely with the sum of resistances in the renal vasculature.

3. GFR varies with the net filtration pressure and capillary filtration coefficient.

Net filtration pressure is determined by renal artery pressure, resistances in the afferent and efferent arterioles, and plasma oncotic pressure.

The kidney has autoregulatory mechanisms that blunt changes in blood flow and GFR in response to changes in renal artery pressure.

STUDY QUESTIONS

2–1. A substance X is known to be freely filtered. Therefore, all of the X that enters the glomerular capillaries is filtered. True or false?

2–2. The concentration of glucose in plasma is 100 mg/dL, and the GFR is 125 mL/min. How much glucose is filtered per minute?

2–3. The concentration of calcium in Bowman's capsule is 3 mEq/L, whereas its plasma concentration is 5 mEq/L. Why are the concentrations different?

2–4. A protein has a molecular weight of 30,000 and a plasma concentration of 100 mg/L. The GFR is 100 L/day. How much of this protein is filtered per day?

2–5. A drug is noted to cause a decrease in GFR. Identify 4 possible actions of the drug that might decrease GFR.

2–6. A drug is noted to cause an increase in GFR with no change in net filtration pressure. What might the drug be doing?

2–7. A person is given a drug that dilates the afferent arteriole and constricts the efferent arteriole by the same amounts. Assuming no other actions of the drug, what happens to this person's GFR, RBF, and filtration fraction?

2–8. A clamp around the renal artery is partially tightened to reduce renal arterial pressure from a mean of 120 to 80 mm Hg. How much do you predict RBF will change?

A. 33% decrease

B. Zero

C. 5–10% decrease

D. 33% increase

Clearance

3

OBJECTIVES

The student understands the principles and applications of clearance technique.

▶ *Defines the terms* clearance *and* metabolic clearance rate, *and differentiates between general clearance and renal clearance.*

▶ *Lists the information required for clearance calculation*

▶ *States the criteria that must be met for a substance so that its clearance can be used as a measure of glomerular filtration rate; states which substances are used to measure glomerular filtration rate and effective renal plasma flow.*

▶ *Given data, calculates C_{In}, C_{PAH}, C_{urea}, $C_{glucose}$, C_{Na}.*

▶ *Predicts whether a substance undergoes net reabsorption or net secretion by comparing its clearance with that of inulin or by comparing its rate of filtration with its rate of excretion.*

▶ *Given data, calculates net rate of reabsorption or secretion for any substance.*

▶ *Given data, calculates fractional excretion of any substance.*

▶ *Describes how to estimate glomerular filtration rate from C_{Cr} and describes the limitations.*

▶ *Describes how to use plasma concentrations of urea and creatinine as indicators of changes in glomerular filtration rate.*

One of the crucial functions of the kidneys is to remove metabolic wastes and excess amounts of ingested substances from the blood. Nitrogenous wastes such as urea and creatinine are generated by metabolism and removed from the body by the kidneys. The average excretion rate normally reflects the rate at which these substances are put into the blood by metabolic processes, thus keeping the body in balance for these substances. Other substances, those that are crucial for normal function, including sodium and potassium, enter the body by ingestion and are also removed from the body by the kidneys. These excretion rates parallel ingestion rate in the long term but are altered transiently to reflect other needs, such as the regulation of blood pressure or plasma osmolality.

 Ridding the body of a substance is often called *clearance*. This term in a biomedical context has both a general meaning and a specific renal meaning. The general meaning of clearance is simply that a substance is removed from the blood by any of several mechanisms. For instance, a drug may be cleared by excretion in the urine or the feces, or it may be transformed by the liver and other peripheral tissues to an inactive form. Renal clearance, on the other hand, means that the substance is removed from the blood and *excreted in the urine.*

The *rate* at which something is cleared can be expressed in several different ways. The most obvious is excretion rate. If a substance leaves the body at a certain amount per hour, this is one way to quantify its clearance. The units of excretion rate are the amount leaving the body per time. Another way to quantify the clearance of a substance is by the substance's plasma half-life. The time it takes for the plasma concentration to fall to half of its current value is the plasma half-life, or $t_{1/2}$. The units are time. Still another way, and the one we develop here, places a more specific meaning on the word clearance. Both general clearance and specific renal clearance can be expressed as the *volume of plasma per unit time from which all of a substance is removed.* For general clearance, this is often called the *metabolic clearance rate,* and when specifically referring to clearance performed by the kidneys, it is called *renal clearance.*

CLEARANCE UNITS

The units of clearance are often confusing to the first-time reader, so let us be sure of the meaning. First, the units are *volume per time* (not amount per time). Consider the renal clearance of a substance X. Suppose substance X has a plasma concentration of 1 mg/dL and is excreted in the urine at a rate of 0.5 mg/min. This means that 0.5 mg of substance X must be removed from the blood plasma each minute. In other words, whatever *volume* of plasma contains 0.5 mg of substance X must represent the clearance of substance X each minute. Each deciliter of plasma entering the kidney brings with it 1 mg of substance X. Because 1 dL of plasma contains 1 mg, then 1/2 of 1 dL (50 mL) contains 0.5 mg. The plasma is cleared of substance X at a rate of 50 mL/min (ie, the renal clearance of substance X is 50 mL/min). Again, note the units: volume per time (ie, the volume of plasma from which a substance is completely removed [cleared]).

The general meaning and specific renal meaning of clearance can be illustrated by comparing how the body handles 2 substances with similar-sounding names but very different properties: insulin and inulin. *Insulin* is the familiar pancreatic hormone involved in regulating blood sugar (glucose). It is a protein with a molecular weight of 5.8 kd and is small enough to be freely filtered by the glomerulus. Once in Bowman's space, it moves along with every other filtered substance into the proximal convoluted tubule, where it is largely taken up by endocytosis and degraded into its constituent amino acids. Very little insulin escapes this uptake, and very little of the filtered insulin makes it all the way to the urine. Thus, the kidney takes part in clearing insulin from the blood; however, because so little appears in the urine, the specific *renal* clearance is very low (<1 mL/min). However, the body has additional mechanisms for clearing insulin, and its *metabolic* clearance rate is quite high (half-life less than 10 min). Let us contrast this with inulin. *Inulin* is a polysaccharide starch of about 5-kd molecular weight. Like insulin, it is freely filtered by the glomerulus, but it is not taken up or transported by the nephron. All the inulin that is filtered flows through the nephron and appears in the urine. Thus, inulin's renal clearance is relatively large. Inulin in the blood is not taken up by other tissues, and the kidneys are the only excretion route. As we will see, this makes inulin a very special substance with respect to assessing renal function.

Quantification of Clearance

Consider again a substance X that is excreted in the urine.

How do we actually calculate clearance in the proper units? The amount excreted must exist in some volume of urine, and that amount must have been contained in some volume of plasma. Those volumes are shown as boxes in Figure 3–1. The small box on the right side of Figure 3–1 represents the volume of urine produced in 1 h (50 mL, or 0.5 dL). The larger box on the left represents the volume of plasma that contained the amount excreted. It is the volume cleared of X. How much X is excreted in 1 h? It is the product of urine concentration of X (U_x) and urine flow rate (V) (ie, 60 mg/dL × 0.5 dL/h = 30 mg/h). That same 30 mg/h cleared from the plasma is also a product of a plasma volume and concentration. Because the plasma concentration (P_x) is 1 mg/dL, it must have required 30 dL of plasma to supply it (ie, the plasma volume cleared in 3–1 h, the clearance of substance X (C_x), must be 30 dL/h. These relationships are shown as numbers in Figure 3–1, Equation 3-1, and symbolically in Figure 3–1, Equation 3-1a. Finally, how do we conveniently calculate the value for C_x? If we divide each side of Equation 3-1 by P_x, we arrive at C_x (shown numerically in Equation 3-2 and symbolically in Equation 3-2a). In other

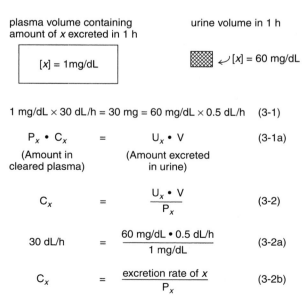

plasma volume containing amount of x excreted in 1 h

urine volume in 1 h

$[x] = 1\,mg/dL$

$[x] = 60\,mg/dL$

$$1\ mg/dL \times 30\ dL/h = 30\ mg = 60\ mg/dL \times 0.5\ dL/h \quad (3\text{-}1)$$

$$P_x \bullet C_x = U_x \bullet V \quad (3\text{-}1a)$$

(Amount in cleared plasma)   (Amount excreted in urine)

$$C_x = \frac{U_x \bullet V}{P_x} \quad (3\text{-}2)$$

$$30\ dL/h = \frac{60\ mg/dL \bullet 0.5\ dL/h}{1\ mg/dL} \quad (3\text{-}2a)$$

$$C_x = \frac{\text{excretion rate of } x}{P_x} \quad (3\text{-}2b)$$

Figure 3–1. Derivation of the basic clearance formula.

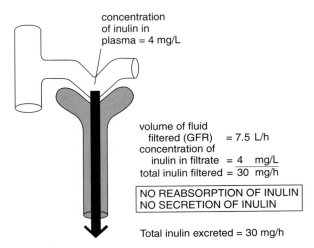

concentration
of inulin in
plasma = 4 mg/L

volume of fluid
   filtered (GFR)   = 7.5 L/h
concentration of
   inulin in filtrate = 4   mg/L
total inulin filtered = 30 mg/h

| NO REABSORPTION OF INULIN |
| NO SECRETION OF INULIN |

Total inulin excreted = 30 mg/h

Figure 3–2. Renal handling of inulin, a substance that is filterable but is neither reabsorbed nor secreted. Therefore, the mass of inulin excreted per unit time is equal to the mass filtered during the same time period. Therefore, as explained in the text, the clearance of inulin is equal to the glomerular filtration rate.

words, *the clearance of substance X is the urine flow rate times the urine concentration of X divided by the plasma concentration of X.* While we are addressing the quantification of clearance, note that the product of urine flow rate and urine concentration is excretion rate. Therefore, we can also state that *the clearance of substance X is the excretion rate divided by the plasma concentration* (Figure 3–1, Equation 3-2b).

Let us now examine the clearance of several substances that are important for the quantification of renal function, starting with inulin.

Inulin, as described previously, is a polysaccharide that is freely filtered and neither reabsorbed nor secreted. All that is filtered is excreted. Therefore, the volume of plasma cleared per unit time is the same as the glomerular filtration rate (GFR) (Figure 3–2). Inulin clearance is indeed the hallmark method of measuring the GFR. Why is inulin so good in this regard? The first property is its filterability. It moves into Bowman's space in the same proportion as the volume filtered. Second, it cannot move in either direction by the paracellular route around the tubular epithelium. The tight junctions are too restrictive to permit saccharides of any sort to move through them. Third, there are no transport mechanisms either on the apical or basolateral surface of the tubular epithelium to take up inulin. Finally, there are no enzymes (amylases) present in the tubular lumen to break down inulin. Thus, it is freely filtered, and all that is filtered moves through the nephron into the urine.

Can something have a clearance *greater* than the GFR? Indeed, yes. One such substance is para-aminohippurate (PAH).

This is a small (molecular weight of 194 D) water-soluble organic anion that is freely filtered and also avidly secreted by the proximal tubule epithelium (via the transcellular route). The secretion rate is saturable. (That is, there is a maximum rate of PAH secretion into the tubule. Such tubular maximum, or T_m, transport systems are common; see Chapter 4.) However, at low plasma concentrations, about 90% of the PAH entering the kidney is removed from the plasma and excreted in the urine. Its clearance, therefore, is nearly as great as the renal plasma flow. In fact, the PAH clearance is used as a measure of renal plasma flow, usually called the *effective renal plasma flow* to indicate that its value is slightly less than the true renal plasma flow.

So far the freely filtered substances we have discussed have clearance values lying between the GFR and the renal plasma flow. Can a freely filtered substance have a clearance value *less* than the GFR? Yes. In fact, many freely filtered substances have clearance values of zero! If a filtered substance is completely removed from the nephron by reabsorption or degradation, then none appears in the urine, and the clearance is zero. We have already seen one example of this: insulin, which is all degraded. Another is glucose, which is normally all reabsorbed.

Many freely filtered substances have clearance values less than the GFR but greater than zero (eg, sodium, chloride, and urea). On occasion, some freely filtered substances have a clearance greater than the GFR (eg, PAH and potassium). What can the clearance of a substance tell us? If we know the GFR (as assessed from inulin clearance) and the clearance of a given substance, then any difference between clearance and GFR represents net secretion or reabsorption (or, in a few rare cases, renal synthesis). If the clearance of a substance exactly equals the GFR, then there has been no *net* reabsorption or secretion. If the clearance is greater than the GFR, there must have been net secretion. Finally, if the clearance is less than the GFR, there must have been net reabsorption. The word *net* in this description is important. As we will see, a number of substances are reabsorbed in certain regions of the nephron and secreted in other regions. The net result of these processes is the sum of everything that happens along the nephron.

To illustrate these concepts, let us look at potassium clearance. Potassium is a small, freely filtered ion. About 70% of the filtered load is reabsorbed in the proximal tubule, and another 20% or so is reabsorbed in the loop of Henle. The rest of the nephron has mechanisms to both secrete and reabsorb potassium. Under some conditions (eg, when potassium ingestion is low), reabsorption dominates, reducing the excretion of potassium and thus its clearance. In other conditions (eg, after ingesting large amounts of potassium in citrus fruit), secretion dominates. In this case, not only is the previously reabsorbed amount secreted back into the tubule, but additional potassium is secreted. The result is that more potassium is excreted than is filtered, and potassium clearance is greater than the GFR.

A Practical Method of Measuring GFR: Creatinine Clearance

The gold standard for measuring GFR is the inulin clearance, as described previously, and this method is used in research studies when an accurate value is needed. The method is cumbersome, however, because inulin must be infused, and it must be infused at a rate sufficient to keep its plasma concentration constant during the period of urine formation and collection. If GFR is normal, between 2.5% and 3.5% of plasma inulin is removed every minute and must be replaced by infusion if GFR is to be accurately determined. For routine assessment of GFR of hospitalized patients, there is an easier method: creatinine clearance. Creatinine is an end product of creatine metabolism and is exported into our blood continuously by skeletal muscle. The rate is proportional to skeletal muscle mass, and to the extent that muscle mass is constant in a given individual, the creatinine production is constant. Creatinine is freely filtered and not reabsorbed. A small amount, however, is secreted by the proximal tubule. Therefore, the creatinine appearing in the urine represents both a filtered component and a secreted component. Because of the secretion, creatinine clearance is slightly higher than the GFR. The secreted fraction is normally about 10% to 20%, so the measured creatinine clearance overestimates GFR by the same percentage. For routine assessment of GFR, this degree of error is acceptable. How does one measure creatinine clearance? Usually, a patient's urine is collected for 24 h, and a blood sample is taken sometime during the collection period. Blood and urine are assayed for creatinine concentration, and we apply the clearance formula (Figure 3–1, Equation 3-2) to yield creatinine clearance. Additional errors cloud the issue (eg, errors in the assays for plasma and urine creatinine concentration or drug-induced alteration of creatinine secretion), so the method is not perfect. For a patient with a very low GFR, the secreted component is a relatively larger fraction of the total amount excreted; therefore, the creatinine clearance more severely overestimates GFR in patients with a very low GFR than in those with normal GFR values. Nevertheless, because of low cost and convenience, creatinine clearance continues to be the most common method for routine assessment of patient GFR.

PLASMA CREATININE AND UREA CONCENTRATIONS AS INDICATORS OF GFR CHANGES

Although creatinine clearance is a valuable clinical determinant of GFR, in practice it is far more common to measure plasma creatinine alone and to use this as an *indicator* of GFR. This approach is justified by the fact that most excreted creatinine gains entry to the tubule by filtration. If we ignore the small amount secreted, there should be an excellent inverse correlation between plasma creatinine concentration and GFR (Figure 3–3).

A normal person's plasma creatinine concentration is about 1 mg/dL. It remains stable because each day the amount of creatinine produced is excreted. Suppose one day the GFR suddenly decreases by 50% because of a blood clot in the renal artery. On that day the person filters only 50% as much creatinine as normal so that creatinine excretion is also reduced by 50%. (We are ignoring the small contribution of secreted creatinine.) Therefore, assuming no change in creatinine production, the person goes into positive creatinine balance, and the plasma creatinine rises. However, despite the persistent 50% GFR reduction, the plasma creatinine does not continue to rise indefinitely; rather, it stabilizes at 2 mg/dL (ie, after it has doubled). At this point, the person once again is able to excrete creatinine at the normal rate and so goes back in balance with a stable plasma level. The reason is that the 50% GFR

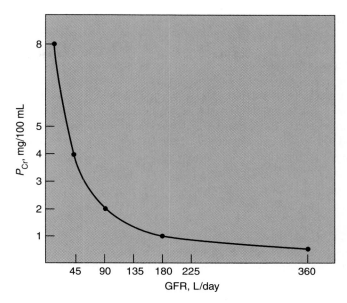

Figure 3–3. Steady-state relationship between GFR and plasma creatine, assuming no creatinine is secreted.

reduction has been just offset by the doubling of plasma creatinine concentration, restoring the filtered load of creatinine to normal. To understand this point, assume an original daily filtration volume of 180 L (1800 dL).

> Original normal state:
> Filtered creatinine = 1 mg/dL × 1800 dL/day = 1800 mg/day
>
> New steady-steady state:
> Filtered creatinine = 2 mg/dL × 900 dL/day = 1800 mg/day

This is a very important point: In the new steady state, creatinine excretion is normal (the person is *in balance*) because of the doubling of plasma creatinine concentration. In other words, creatinine excretion is below normal only *transiently* until plasma creatinine has increased as much proportionally as the GFR has fallen.

What if the GFR then fell to 300 dL/day? Again, creatinine retention would occur until a new steady state had been established (ie, until the person was again filtering 1800 mg/day). What would the new plasma creatinine be?

$$1800 \text{ mg/day} = P_{Cr} \times 300 \text{ dL/day}$$
$$P_{Cr} = 6 \text{ mg/dL}$$

The rise in plasma creatinine results directly from the fall in GFR. Therefore, a single plasma creatinine measurement is a reasonable *indicator* of GFR. It is not completely accurate, however, for several reasons: (1) As before, some creatinine is secreted; (2) there is no way of knowing exactly what the person's original creatinine was when GFR was normal; (3) creatinine production may not remain completely unchanged. However, a *rising* plasma creatinine is a red flag that there may be a renal problem.

Because urea is also handled by filtration, the same type of analysis suggests that the measurement of plasma urea concentration could also serve as an indicator of GFR. However, it is a much less accurate indicator than plasma creatinine because the range of normal plasma urea concentration varies widely, depending on protein intake and changes in tissue catabolism, and because urea excretion is under partial hormonal regulation.

KEY CONCEPTS

 Clearance has both a general meaning describing loss of material from the body and a specific renal meaning involving the kidney's ability to remove substances from the blood. Renal clearance is always expressed in units of volume per time.

 Renal clearance of any substance X is quantified by a general clearance formula relating urine flow to urine and plasma concentrations:

$$C_X = \frac{U_X}{P_X} \bullet V$$

 Inulin clearance is used to measure GFR because inulin is freely filtered and neither secreted nor reabsorbed.

 Para-aminohippurate clearance is used as a practical estimate of renal blood flow.

 Creatinine clearance is used as practical estimate of GFR.

 STUDY QUESTIONS

3–1. *The hospital lab reports that your patient's creatinine clearance is 120 g/day. This value is*

A. *Normal*

B. *Significantly below normal*

C. *Not an interpretable number as presented*

3–2. A substance is known to be cleared from the body both by renal excretion and by nonrenal mechanisms. Is the renal clearance higher, lower, or the same as the metabolic clearance rate?

3–3. An increase in the plasma concentration of inulin during infusion causes which of the following in the renal clearance of inulin?

A. Increase

B. Decrease

C. No change

3–4. The clearance of substance A is less than that simultaneously determined for inulin. Give 3 possible explanations.

3–5. The clearance of substance B is greater than the simultaneously determined clearance for inulin. What is the possible explanation for this?

3–6. List, in order of decreasing renal clearance, the following substances: glucose, urea, sodium, inulin, creatinine, PAH.

3–7. The following test results were obtained during a clearance experiment:

$U_{In} = 50\ mg/L$

$P_{In} = 1\ mg/L$

$V = 2\ mL/min$

$U_{Na} = 75\ mmol/L$

$P_{Na} = 150\ mmol/L$

What is the fractional excretion of sodium?

3–8. A month after 80% of the nephrons are destroyed, what will the blood urea concentration be, assuming it was 5 mmol/L before the disease occurred and assuming dietary protein remains the same?

A. 25 mmol/L

B. 5 mmol/L

C. 6 mmol/L

D. Continuously rising

Basic Transport Mechanisms

OBJECTIVES

The student understands the basic mechanisms of tubular reabsorption and secretion:

▶ Defines and states the major characteristics of diffusion, facilitated diffusion, primary active transport, secondary active transport (including symport and antiport) and endocytosis.

▶ Describes the major morphological components of an epithelial tissue, including lumen, serosa, interstitium, apical and basolateral membranes, tight junctions, and lateral spaces.

▶ States how the mechanisms listed in Objective 1 can be combined to achieve active transcellular reabsorption in epithelial tissues.

▶ Defines paracellular transport and differentiates between transcellular and paracellular transport.

▶ Defines osmolality and osmolarity, and states why osmolarity is commonly used to approximate osmolality.

▶ Describes what is meant by the expression "water follows the osmoles."

▶ Describes qualitatively the forces that determine movement of reabsorbed fluid from the interstitium into peritubular capillaries.

▶ Compares the Starling forces governing glomerular filtration with those governing peritubular capillary absorption.

▶ Compares and contrasts the concepts of T_m and gradient-limited transport.

▶ Describes 3 processes that can produce bidirectional transport of a substance in a single tubular segment; states the consequences of pump-leak systems.

▶ Contrasts "tight" and "leaky" epithelia.

The basic processes of tubular reabsorption and secretion first mentioned in Chapter 1 involve crossing 2 barriers: the tubular epithelium and the endothelial cells lining the peritubular capillaries. (For the moment, we are leaving aside substances that are synthesized or degraded by the renal epithelium.) For reabsorbed substances, the endothelial cell barrier of the peritubular capillaries is like the barrier of many other peripheral capillary beds in the body: Solutes cross the peritubular capillary barrier through the basement membrane and then the fenestrae in the endothelial cells. For secreted substances, crossing the endothelium is similar to the filtration process in the glomerular capillaries, but it is going "upstream" in the sense that *volume* is moving from interstitium to capillary (as part of the tubular reabsorptive process), whereas the secreted substance is traveling in the opposite direction. However, because the endothelium is highly permeable to small solutes, this is quite feasible providing there is a suitable concentration gradient.

CROSSING THE EPITHELIAL BARRIERS

Crossing the epithelium lining the tubule can be done in a single step or 2 steps. The *paracellular* route (single step) is when the substance goes *around* the cells (ie, through the matrix of the tight junctions that link each epithelial cell to its neighbor (Figure 4–1). More often, however, the substance goes *through* the cells, a 2-step process: across the apical membrane facing the tubular lumen and across the basolateral membrane facing the interstitium. This is called the *transcellular* route.

An array of mechanisms exists by which substances cross the various barriers. The general classes of mechanisms are no different from those used elsewhere in the body to transport substances across cell membranes. We can view these mechanisms as a physiological tool box. Renal cells use whichever set of tools is most suitable for the task. The general classes of mechanisms for traversing the barriers are depicted in Figure 4–2.

Movement by Diffusion

Diffusion is the frenzied random movement of free molecules in solution (like the Ping-Pong balls in a lottery drawing). *Net diffusion* occurs across a barrier (ie, more molecules moving one way than the other) if there is driving force (a concentration gradient or, for charged molecules, a potential gradient) and if the barrier is permeable. This applies to almost all substances crossing the endothelial barrier lining the peritubular capillaries. It applies to substances taking the paracellular route around the tubular epithelium and to some substances taking the transcellular route through membranes. Substances that are lipid soluble, such as the blood gases or steroids, can diffuse directly through the lipid bilayer.

Movement Through Channels

Most substances that are biologically important cannot penetrate lipid membranes. To cross a membrane, they must move through specific integral membrane proteins, which are divided into categories of *channels* and *transporters* (see Figure 4–2). Channels are small pores (proteins with a "channel" or pathway through the interior of the protein) that permit, depending on their structure, water or specific solutes to diffuse through them. Thus, we use the terms *sodium channel* and *potassium channel* to designate channels that permit diffusion of these molecular species. Aquaporins are channels selectively permeable to water. Movement through channels is passive (ie, no external energy is required). The energy to drive the diffusion is inherent in the concentration gradient or, strictly speaking, the electrochemical gradient, because ions are driven through channels and around cells via the paracellular route not only by gradients of concentration but also by gradients

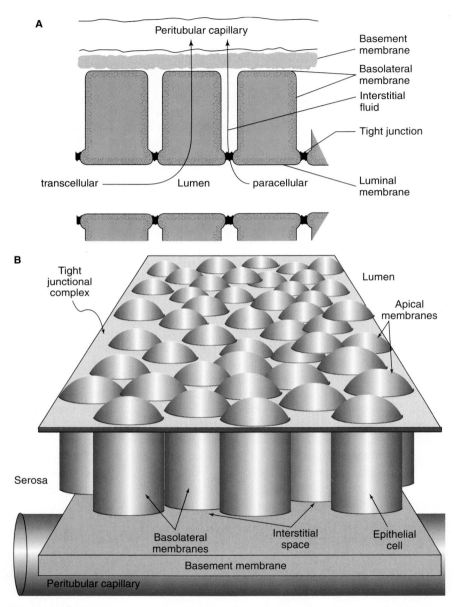

Figure 4–1. Diagrammatic representation of tubular epithelium. The tight junctions can be visualized three dimensionally as the sheet of plastic holding together a six-pack of soda, each cell being one of the cans.

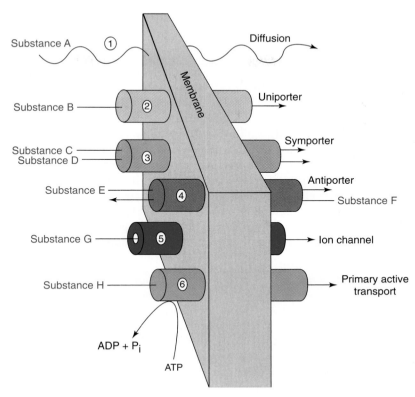

Figure 4–2. Basic mechanisms of transmembrane solute transport. See text for details.

of voltage. Channels represent a mechanism for rapidly moving across membranes large amounts of specific substances, which would otherwise diffuse slowly or not at all. The amount of material passing through an ion channel can be controlled by opening and closing the channel pore.

Movement by Transporters

Our genome codes for a large array of proteins that function as transporters, all with names and acronyms that suffuse the physiological literature. Transporters, like channels, permit the transmembrane flux of a solute that is otherwise impermeable in the lipid bilayer. Channels can move large amounts of materials across membranes in a short period of time, but in many cases, they do not distinguish well among substances they transport; that is, their specificity is often relatively low. However, unlike channels, many transporters are extremely specific, transporting only 1 or at most a small class of substances. On the other hand, the specificity is also usually coupled to a lower rate of transport because the transported solutes bind much more strongly to the transport protein. Furthermore, the protein must undergo a more elaborate cycle of conformational change to move the solute from one side of the membrane to the other. To avoid unnecessary complexity, we can group transporters into categories according to basic functional properties.

UNIPORTERS

Uniporters permit movement of a single solute species through the membrane. The basic difference between a channel and a uniporter is that a channel is a tiny hole, whereas a uniporter requires that the solute bind to a site that is alternately available to one side and then the other side of the membrane (like entering a vestibule through an outside door and then leaving the vestibule to enter a hallway through an inside door). Movement through a uniporter is often called *facilitated diffusion* because, like diffusion, it is driven by concentration gradients, but the transported material moves through the uniporter protein rather than the membrane. A set of uniporters crucial for all cells includes those that facilitate the movement of glucose across cell membranes. These are members of the GLUT family of proteins that permit, in the kidney's proximal tubule epithelial cells, glucose to move from the cytosol across the basolateral membrane into the interstitium.

SYMPORTERS AND ANTIPORTERS

Symporters and *antiporters* move 2 or more solute species in the same direction across a membrane (symporters) or in opposite directions across a membrane (antiporters). In the literature, transport by a symporter is sometimes called *cotransport,* whereas transport by an antiporter is called *exchange or counter transport.* Thus, there are symporters that move sodium and glucose together into cells (members of the SGLT protein family) and symporters that move sodium, potassium, and chloride all together into a cell. In the case of the SGLT family, each transport cycle moves 1 glucose molecule and either 1 or 2 sodium ions depending on the particular SGLT. There are antiporters that move sodium into a cell and protons out of a cell (often called sodium-hydrogen exchangers, members of the NHE protein family). Another key antiporter in many cells, including the kidney, moves chloride in one direction and bicarbonate in the opposite direction.

All molecular transport requires energy. In the case of diffusion through a channel or movement via a uniporter, the energy is inherent in the electrochemical gradient for the solute. With symporters and antiporters, at least 1 of the solutes moves down its electrochemical gradient and provides the energy to move 1 or more of the other solutes up its electrochemical gradient. Movement of any solute up its electrochemical gradient is called *active transport.* In the case of symporters and antiporters that do not hydrolyze ATP, the active transport is called *secondary* active transport because the energy is provided indirectly from the transport of another solute rather than directly from a chemical reaction. In a large number of cases, sodium is one of the solutes moved by a symporter or antiporter to provide energy. The energetics of sodium distribution always favors entrance (eg, if a sodium channel exists, sodium will enter, not leave, the cell). When sodium movement is coupled to that of another solute, as in sodium-proton antiport (exchange), sodium will enter passively, and the other solute will move in the opposite direction actively *if* the energy obtained from moving sodium down its electrochemical gradient is greater than that required to move the other solute up its gradient. The stochiometry is important here. The energy available from a gradient is multiplied by the number of molecules that move per transport cycle. For example, some SGLT proteins move 2 sodium ions per transport cycle; others move only 1. There is more energy available to actively transport glucose through an SGLT protein that moves 2 sodium ions than one that transports 1 sodium ion per glucose. Another example is the coupled transport of bicarbonate and sodium. An important symporter in the proximal tubule is a so-called NBCe transporter, which moves 3 bicarbonate ions and 1 sodium ion per transport cycle. The electrochemical gradient for bicarbonate is directly outward, and the energy gained from moving 3 bicarbonate ions outward is greater than the energy it takes to move 1 sodium ion outward. Therefore, this transporter moves these solutes outward, *up* the electrochemical gradient for sodium.

PRIMARY ACTIVE TRANSPORTERS

Primary active transporters are membrane proteins that are capable of moving 1 or more solutes up their electrochemical gradients, using the energy obtained from the hydrolysis of adenosine triphosphate (ATP). All transporters that move solutes in this manner are ATPases (ie, their structure is both that of an enzyme that splits ATP and a transporter that has binding sites that alternately are open to one side and then the other side of the membrane). Among the key primary active transporters in the kidney is the ubiquitous Na-K-ATPase (often called the "sodium pump"), some isoform of which is present in all cells of the body. This transporter simultaneously moves sodium against its electrochemical gradient out of a cell and potassium against its gradient into a cell. The stochiometry is 3 sodium ions out and 2 potassium ions for every ATP molecule hydrolyzed. Other crucial primary active transport systems are a set of H-ATPases, which move protons out of cells, and Ca-ATPases, which move calcium out of cells. All of these ATPases belong to a large family of homologous transporter proteins.

RECEPTOR-MEDIATED ENDOCYTOSIS AND TRANSCYTOSIS

Almost all the secretion and reabsorption of solutes discussed throughout this textbook use some combination of the just-mentioned set of membrane permeability mechanisms. One other solute transport process of some importance is *receptor-mediated endocytosis.* In this case, a solute, usually a protein, binds to a site on the apical surface of an epithelial cell, and then a patch of membrane with the solute bound to it is internalized as a vesicle in the cytoplasm. Subsequent processes then degrade the protein into its constituent amino acids, which are transported across the basolateral membrane and into the blood.

For a few proteins, particularly immunoglobulins, endocytosis can occur at either the apical or basolateral membranes, after which the endocytic vesicles remain intact and are transported to the opposite cellular membrane, where they undergo exocytosis to release the protein intact. Such *transcytosis* is very important in the host defense mechanisms of the kidney and in the prevention of urinary tract infections.

Hydrostatic Flow, Osmosis, and Osmotic Pressure

Hydrostatic pressure (hydraulic pressure) drives the volume flux of filtration across the endothelial walls of glomerular capillaries (the filtration process described in

Chapter 2). We described the role of plasma proteins in generating an oncotic pressure that opposed filtration. We now discuss their role a little further, along with the general role of solutes in controlling volume flux across a barrier.

 As long as solutes are equally permeable as water, they will move along with filtered water or reabsorbed water and have the same concentration in the filtrate as in the plasma. Solutes play a different role when a barrier (epithelial layer or cell membrane) is less permeable to solutes than to water.

Solutes dissolved in water reduce the concentration of water and, therefore, reduce the tendency of water to diffuse out of a solution. Solutions that are highly concentrated with solutes are lower in *water* concentration. Therefore, when solutions of different solute concentration are separated by a barrier, water will move from the more dilute solution to the more concentrated solution (ie, from where the *water* is more concentrated to where the *water* is less concentrated). This process is called *osmosis*. The ability of solutes to lower the concentration of water is called *osmolality*. It is a function both of the *concentration* of solutes and the *kind* of solutes. For example, proteins are better than sugars, and sugars are better than small ions, at lowering the concentration of water.

Osmolality is expressed in units of osmoles per kilogram of water (or, more commonly, milliosmoles per kilogram). Osmolality is often called *osmotic pressure.*

Osmolality and osmotic pressure have the same meaning; they are just expressed in different units (1 mOsm/kg = 19.3 mm Hg of osmotic pressure). To say that a solution has a high osmotic pressure means that it has a high osmolality. Given a cell membrane or epithelial layer in which the solutions on the 2 sides have different osmolalities, water will move by osmosis *toward* the side with the higher osmolality. A convenient way to express this is to say that "water follows the osmoles."

Now for a crucial point: Osmolality (osmotic pressure) is only effective in driving osmosis when the barrier is less permeable to solutes than to water. (Imagine a barrier made of chicken wire. Regardless of solute concentrations, there would be no osmosis because there would be no restriction on the diffusion of solute.) In the endothelial barriers of glomerular capillaries and peritubular capillaries, most of the solutes are as permeable through the fenestrae as water and thus do not influence water movement. However, the large plasma proteins are not permeable, and they do indeed influence water movement. The osmotic pressure resulting from the proteins only (ignoring everything else) is called the *colloid osmotic pressure* or *oncotic pressure.* Colloid osmotic pressure is a component of the Starling forces governing filtration and absorption across endothelial layers. In other barriers, specifically the epithelial lining of the renal tubules, solute permeabilities are generally lower than water permeability. Therefore, all solutes contribute to driving a water flux. Here, *all* of the osmolality, not just the component resulting from proteins, is important.

Knowing the osmolality of a solution is impossible without measuring it (it cannot be calculated even if we know the concentrations of everything in the solution. For some solutes, we can consult tables and then interpolate between table values. For most solutes, no such tables exist.) However, we can get a rough idea of the osmolality or "guesstimate" it from a related quantity called the *osmolarity.* The osmolarity is simply the sum of the molar concentrations of all solutes without regard to kind. Osmolarity is expressed in units of osmoles per liter (or usually milliosmoles per liter). A solution containing 140 mEq/L of sodium, 140 mEq/L of chloride, and 10 mmol/L glucose has an osmolarity of 190 mOsm/L (140 + 140 + 10 = 190).

Fortunately, when osmol*ality* is measured (milliosmoles per kilogram of water) and osmol*arity* is calculated from solution ingredients (milliosmoles per liter), the results are usually within 10% of each other. For convenience, physiologists often calculate osmolarity and then *call it* osmolality, and accept the error in this calculation as the price paid for convenience.

The difference between osmolality and osmolarity is illustrated in the case of physiological saline (0.9% NaCl, or 154 mmol/L NaCl). This solution is commonly used as a hospital infusion solution because it matches the normal osmolality of human plasma (280–290 mOsm/kg). The osmolarity of this solution is 154 + 154 = 308 mOsm/L, but when measured, the osmolality is 287 mOsm/kg.

TRANSPORT MECHANISMS IN REABSORPTION

Quantitatively, most of the transport in the kidney consists of reabsorption. Virtually all of the 180 L of water and several pounds of salt that are filtered each day into Bowman's space in the glomeruli must be reabsorbed, along with large amounts of many other substances. Much of the reabsorption is *iso-osmotic,* meaning that water and solutes are reabsorbed in equal proportions. Recall that filtration in the glomerulus is iso-osmotic. Almost all solutes (except large plasma proteins) move from plasma into the filtrate in the same proportion as water; thus, their concentration in the glomerular filtrate is the same as in the plasma. In the proximal tubule, where the majority of reabsorption occurs, the process is virtually iso-osmotic. In the later portions of the nephron, reabsorption is generally not iso-osmotic (a point that is crucial for our ability to separately regulate solute and water balance).

Most of the solute reabsorbed in the proximal tubule consists of sodium and the anions that must accompany the sodium to maintain electroneutrality: mostly chloride and bicarbonate. These solutes are removed from the tubular lumen and put into the interstitium by a combination of the processes described previously. Thus, a large amount of solute is transferred from lumen to interstitium, setting up an osmotic gradient that favors the parallel movement of water. The proximal tubule epithelium is very permeable to water, and water—a substantial amount—indeed follows solute from the lumen to the interstitium. The water moves in equal proportions as solute, so that both the fluid removed from the lumen and that remaining behind are essentially iso-osmotic with the original filtrate (ie, have the same osmolality). We say "essentially" because there must be *some* difference in osmolality to induce water movement, but for an epithelial barrier (like the proximal tubule) that is very permeable to water, a difference of 1 mOsm/kg or less is sufficient to drive reabsorption of water.

Tubular hydrostatic pressure is several millimeters of mercury greater than interstitial hydrostatic pressure, and this pressure gradient also favors reabsorption. However, under normal circumstances, this is a small influence. It requires a hydrostatic pressure gradient of 19.3 mm Hg to act as an equivalent driving force as an osmotic gradient of 1 mOsm/kg, and the hydrostatic pressure difference is usually not more than 5–8 mm Hg.

Once in the interstitium, the solutes and water move from interstitium into the peritubular capillaries and are returned to the systemic circulation. Otherwise, the kidney would swell without limit.

Fortunately, the Starling forces across the peritubular capillaries favor reabsorption. The capillary hydraulic pressure, which was about 60 mm Hg in the glomerular capillaries, has fallen to about 15–20 mm Hg, and the plasma oncotic pressure, resulting from filtration in the glomerular capillaries, has risen to more than 30 mm Hg (Table 4–1). Therefore, the net filtration pressure is now a net absorptive pressure, and fluid is reabsorbed back into the peritubular capillaries. The alert student can appreciate the fact that if cortical Starling forces are abnormal (eg, low plasma oncotic pressure as when liver disease prevents normal production of serum albumin), absorption of fluid from the cortical interstitium can be slowed, causing a backup of fluid that inhibits fluid movement from tubular lumen to interstitium. Ultimately, this can lead to increased excretion from the body.

As blood flows through the peritubular capillaries, there is rapid diffusion of individual molecules back and forth between capillary plasma and interstitial fluid. The total volume of interstitial space is only 4% of the total cortical volume, and the vascular volume is a little higher. Given the very high renal blood flow, the solute concentrations in the interstitial fluid are essentially clamped to those in the blood perfusing the cortex. The cortical interstitium remains quite plasma like (minus the proteins) in its composition, even though large amounts of solute continuously cross through the interstitium from tubule to blood.

With all of these factors as a background, let us more closely examine how things are reabsorbed. We can take an anthropomorphic view and ask, "If I'm a molecule

Table 4–1. Estimated forces involved in movement of fluid from interstitium into peritubular capillaries*

Forces		mm Hg
1	Favoring uptake	
	a Interstitial hydraulic pressure, P_{Int}	3
	b Oncotic pressure in peritubular capillaries, π_{PC}	33
2	Opposing uptake	
	a Hydraulic pressure in peritubular capillaries, P_{PC}	20
	b Interstitial oncotic pressure, π_{Int}	6
3	Net pressure for uptake (1 – 2)	10

* The values for peritubular-capillary hydraulic and oncotic pressures are for the early portions of the capillary. The oncotic pressure, of course, decreases as protein-free fluid enters it (ie, as absorption occurs) but would not go below 25 mm Hg (the value of arterial plasma) even if all fluid originally filtered at the glomerulus were absorbed.

in the lumen, what induces me to go across the epithelial layer instead of just staying where I am?"

Generalized Epithelial Transport: The Transcellular Route

Epithelial transport requires that epithelial cells are *polarized* (ie, the proteins present in the apical and the basolateral membrane are not the same). This polarization can promote net flux of sodium from lumen to serosa, which is the linchpin around which the transport of virtually every other substance depends. Figure 4–3 shows the morphology of a generalized renal epithelium in which salt and water transport can be viewed as a 4-step process. Step 1 is the active extrusion of sodium via Na-K-ATPase from the cell to the serosa (interstitium). This creates a low concentration of sodium within the cell so that sodium moves downhill from the lumen to the cell interior via a variety of symporters, antiporters, and channels. A key player in the proximal tubule is the sodium-proton antiporter (NHE-3 isoform) that we discuss further later. The consequence of this transcellular sodium movement is separation of charge (excess Na^+ on the serosal side) that promotes Step 2, the movement of anions to balance the positive charge. The accumulation of sodium and anions in the interstitial space produces an osmotic gradient from lumen to serosa that

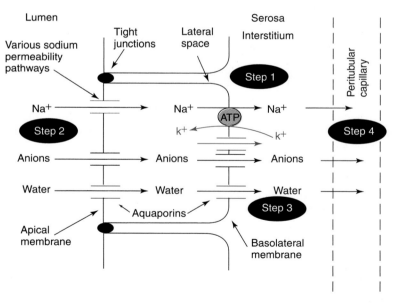

Figure 4–3. Steps involved in transporting solute and water from the tubular lumen to the peritubular capillary. Everything depends on and follows logically from Step 1, which is the active extrusion of sodium into the interstitium. This induces a parallel transport of anions (Step 2). The movement of sodium and anions generates an osmotic drive that causes reabsorption of water (Step 3). Finally, the increased volume in the interstitium alters peritubular Starling forces and induces the bulk flow of water and solute from interstitium into the peritubular capillary (Step 4).

promotes water movement (Step 3). Finally, the accumulation of salt and water in the interstitium promotes the bulk flow of solute and water into the peritubular capillaries (Step 4) driven by Starling forces (see Table 4–1). In Step 1, any reabsorbed substance that enters the epithelial cells with sodium across the apical membrane must exit across the basolateral membrane. The particular mechanism by which this occurs depends on the substance. For example, we know that glucose exits via a GLUT uniporter. Many other substances also move via their own uniporters. We examine some of these more closely later as we discuss transport mechanisms in individual tubular segments, but, in general, the transcellular route involves crossing 2 membranes—apical and basolateral—and the transporters in the 2 membranes are different.

The Paracellular Route

As water follows sodium and its anions across the epithelium, the volume remaining in the lumen decreases. Therefore, any solute that has not been specifically transported via the transcellular route will become more concentrated. If two thirds of the water is removed, a nontransported solute will increase in concentration to 3 times its original value. As the luminal concentration rises, this generates a concentration gradient across the tight junctions between the lumen and the interstitium. If the tight junctions are permeable to the substance in question ("leaky"), the substance will diffuse from the lumen to the interstitium. This is precisely what happens to many solutes (eg, urea, potassium, chloride, calcium, and magnesium) in the proximal tubule. The exact fractions that are reabsorbed depends on the permeability of the tight junctions but are generally in the range of one half to two thirds. Because ions are driven not only by concentration gradients but also voltage gradients, the transepithelial voltage plays a role here also. Early in the proximal tubule, the lumen is slightly negative relative to the interstitium (a few millivolts), whereas later it is slightly positive. This voltage enhances paracellular anion reabsorption early and reduces it later. To keep things simple, we can account for most paracellular reabsorption purely on the basis of the rise in luminal concentration that occurs when water is reabsorbed. One substance that does not get reabsorbed by the paracellular route is glucose. First, it is transported by the transcellular route. Second, the tight junctions are not permeable to saccharides. Thus, it cannot diffuse no matter how large the concentration gradient might be.

Limits on Rate of Transport: T_m and Gradient-Limited Systems

Even though the transport capacity of the renal cortex is huge, it is not infinite. There are upper limits to the speed with which any given solute can be reabsorbed from the tubular lumen to capillary blood. In certain situations, these limits are reached, with the consequence that more than the usual amount of solute is not reabsorbed (ie, left in the lumen to be passed on to the next nephron segment). In general, transport mechanisms can be classified by the properties of these limits as either (1) tubular maximum-limited (T_m) systems or (2) gradient-limited systems. T_m systems reach an upper limit because the transporters moving the substance become saturated; any further increase in solute concentration does not increase the rate at which the substance binds to the transporter and thereafter moves through the membrane. Gradient-limited systems reach an upper limit because the tight junctions are leaky, and any significant lowering of luminal concentration relative to the interstitium results in a leak back into the lumen as fast as the substance is transported out. Thus, the limiting rate for the T_m-limited system is a property of the transporter, whereas the limiting rate of a gradient limited system is a property of the permeability of the epithelial monolayer regardless of the maximal rate of the transport protein.

Let us explain T_m-limited systems using glucose as an example. Glucose is present in plasma at a concentration of about 5 mmol/L (90 mg/dL) and is freely filtered. It is reabsorbed by the transcellular route. Glucose enters the epithelial cells across the apical membrane via a symporter with sodium (a member of the SGLT protein family) and exits across the basolateral membrane into the interstitium via a uniporter (a GLUT protein family member). Normally, all the filtered glucose is reabsorbed in the proximal tubule, with none remaining in the lumen to be passed on to the loop of Henle. However, if the filtered load of glucose is abnormally high, the SGLT proteins' upper limit for reabsorbtion is reached. That upper limit is the tubular maximum, or T_m, for glucose. It is the maximum rate at which the substance (glucose in this case) can be reabsorbed regardless of the luminal concentration. Any increase in filtered load above the T_m, which represents a pathological situation, results in glucose being passed on to the loop of Henle. T_m systems are perhaps like snow shovelers keeping a driveway clear during a snowstorm. With an ordinary snowfall, they can remove snow as it falls and keep a driveway clear. However, during a blizzard, snow falls faster than it can be shoveled and accumulates. (Although we are discussing T_m systems in terms of reabsorption, the same concept applies to secretion. For some secreted substances, there is a T_m limit to how fast they are secreted, and a rise in plasma concentration does not increase the secretion rate above the T_m.)

Gradient-limited systems are more complicated than T_m systems. The key to gradient-limited systems is that the epithelium has a finite passive permeability to the substance, usually through the tight junctions, such that a large concentration gradient between the interstitium and lumen results in a large passive flux. Consider the case of sodium. In the proximal tubule, the tight junctions are quite permeable to sodium. Any significant rise in concentration in the interstitium relative to the lumen results in a large passive flux from the interstitium back into the lumen. Sodium is freely filtered and present in the luminal fluid at a concentration of about 140 mEq/L, the same as in plasma. It is reabsorbed by the variety of pathways described previously (ie, symporters and antiporters in the apical membrane and the Na-K-ATPase across the basolateral membrane into the interstitium). As sodium is transported into the interstitium, the interstitial concentration begins to rise. This rise creates a gradient that drives a flux of sodium out of the interstitium, into the peritubular capillaries, and back through the tight junctions into the lumen. Most of the sodium moves into the blood, accomplishing the goal of reabsorption, but some does leak back into the lumen. When the concentration of sodium reaches a sufficiently high level in the interstitium, the concentration gradient between the interstitium and the lumen drives sodium back across the tight junctions as fast as it can be transported through the transcellular pathway from lumen to interstitium. At this point, transport through paracellular and transcellular pathways is large, but *net* transport is zero: The system has established the largest gradient possible, its gradient limit. The leakier the epithelium, the lower is the gradient limit (in the proximal tubule, the gradient limit is about 2 millimolar sodium).

Technically, back-leak of sodium is a secretion, and net sodium reabsorption is the difference between reabsorption from lumen to interstitium and secretion from interstitium to lumen. Because the net transport is indeed reabsorption, we will say simply that sodium is reabsorbed, with a limit placed by the amount of back-leak.

KEY CONCEPTS

Reabsorption is a 2-step process: lumen to interstitium, and interstitium to peritubular capillary.

Flux from lumen to interstitium can be transcellular, *using separate transport steps in the apical and basolateral membranes,* or paracellular, *around the cells through tight junctions.*

Channels and transporters promote the transmembrane flux of solutes that cannot permeate lipid bilayers.

Osmotic gradients drive a volume flux across membranes and epithelia if the solutes are less permeable than water.

Osmotic pressure and osmolality mean the same thing and represent the power of dissolved solute to drive an osmotic flux of water.

For convenience, osmolality is approximated by the easier concept of osmolarity.

Water and solutes, which are reabsorbed from lumen to interstitium, then move from interstitium to peritubular capillaries by bulk flow, driven by Starling forces.

The reabsorption of water and almost all solutes is linked, directly or indirectly, to the active reabsorption of sodium.

All reabsorptive processes have a limit on how fast they can occur, either because the transporters saturate (T_m systems) or because the substance leaks back into the lumen (gradient-limited systems).

STUDY QUESTIONS

4–1.   Flux of a solute out of a cell via a uniporter, symporter, or an ATPase is an example of active transport (primary or secondary). True or false?

4–2.   Reabsorption in the proximal tubule is described as being iso-osmotic, yet we already know from earlier chapters that the excreted urine usually is quite different osmotically from the surrounding interstitium. Why is the final urine not always iso-osmotic?

4–3.   In the proximal tubule, the tubular epithelium is far less permeable to small solutes than is the endothelium of the surrounding peritubular capillaries. True or false?

4–4.   Low plasma oncotic pressure inhibits volume reabsorption from tubular lumen to interstitium. Because this is plasma oncotic pressure, how can it affect trans-epithelial transport?

4–5.   Even though values of osmolality and osmolarity differ numerically, any 2 solutions of equal osmolarity will have equal osmolality. True or false?

4–6.   Given the high volume of fluid normally moving from interstitium to blood in the renal cortex, how can secreted substances move from blood to epithelium? Are they not going the wrong way?

4–7.   The T_m for glucose is set

   A.   Close to the normal filtered load

   B.   Well above the normal filtered load

   C.   Well below the normal filtered load

Renal Handling of Organic Substances

OBJECTIVES

The student understands the renal handling of certain organic substances, specifically including urea:

▶ *States the physiological utility of either excreting or saving organic solutes.*

▶ *States the general characteristics of the proximal tubular systems for active reabsorption or secretion of organic nutrients.*

▶ *Describes the renal handling of glucose and states the conditions under which glucosuria is likely to occur.*

▶ *Describes the renal handling of proteins and small peptides.*

▶ *Describes the secretion of para-aminohippurate.*

▶ *Outlines the handling of urate.*

▶ *Describes the secretion of organic cations.*

▶ *Describes, in general terms, the renal handling of weak acids and bases and how tubular pH affects reabsorption.*

▶ *Describes the renal handling of urea, including the medullary recycling of urea from the collecting duct to the loop of Henle.*

Subsequent chapters of this textbook deal almost exclusively with the renal handling of salt and water and the other major physiological ions in blood because homeostatic regulation of their excretion is of such crucial importance. However, as pointed out in Chapter 1, another major renal function is the excretion of organic waste products, foreign chemicals, and their metabolites. Furthermore, the kidneys filter large amounts of substances that they do not excrete; therefore, reabsorptive processes must exist to prevent inappropriate loss of useful organic nutrients. Because the blood contains many small, filterable molecular species, the kidney has to handle all of them. An analysis of the renal transport pathways for all these organic substances is an overwhelming task, so this chapter briefly describes some of the major pathways. In short, however, the kidney (1) keeps or saves (reabsorbs) organic metabolites that should not be lost and (2) excretes waste products and foreign organic substances to prevent their accumulation.

One organic substance, urea, is unique in this regard. It is a waste product that must be excreted to prevent accumulation. However, it also plays a key role in renal regulation of water balance. We briefly present the renal handling of urea later in this chapter and again in Chapter 6 in the discussion of renal handling of water.

ACTIVE PROXIMAL REABSORPTION OF ORGANIC NUTRIENTS (EG, GLUCOSE, AMINO ACIDS)

Most major cellular nutrients are freely filterable, including glucose, amino acids, acetate, Krebs cycle intermediates, certain water-soluble vitamins, lactate, acetoacetate, β-hydroxybutyrate, and many others. The proximal tubule is the major site for reabsorption of the large quantities of organic nutrients filtered each day by the renal corpuscles. The characteristics of glucose reabsorption described in Chapter 4 are typical of the transport processes for most nutrients. In general,

1. They are actively transported (ie, can be reabsorbed up their respective electrochemical gradients). Indeed, the luminal concentration of the substances in many cases can be reduced virtually to zero (ie, reabsorption can be very close to 100% complete).

2. The "uphill" step is across the luminal membrane, usually via a symporter with sodium.

3. Most are characterized as T_m systems (have an upper limit to the speed at which they can transport). These limits are usually well above the amounts normally filtered. Accordingly, the kidneys return these filtered substances back to the plasma; however, because there is no opportunity to vary the amount excreted (there is none), the kidneys do not help regulate their levels in the body. It is also true, however, that under abnormal conditions the plasma concentration of these substances may increase so much that the filtered load exceeds the reabsorptive T_m and large quantities are excreted in the urine. Examples are glucose, acetoacetate, and β-hydroxybutyrate in patients with severe uncontrolled diabetes.

4. They manifest specificity. This means that a given transporter selectively takes up one or a few substrates and ignores all others. However, there is not a separate transporter for every solute in the body. Two or more closely related substances may use the same transporter. For example, the amino acid transporters are distinct from those for glucose and other monosaccharides, but there are not 20 separate transporters, one for each amino acid. Rather there is one for arginine, lysine, and ornithine; another for glutamate and aspartate; and so on. Shared pathways imply that there is competition among those substances using the same transporter. Practically, this means that an excess of one substance, ornithine for example, in the blood may lead to not only excess ornithine excretion but also inappropriate excretion of arginine and lysine.

5. They are inhibitable by a variety of drugs, and several monogenetic diseases are associated with loss of function in one or more of these proximal reabsorptive systems. In some cases the deficit may be highly specific (eg, involving only one amino acid), whereas in others multiple systems may be involved (eg, glucose and many amino acids). This range of defects is also seen when the deficit is due to an ingested toxin (eg, lead toxicity) rather than a genetic abnormality.

Glucose

Because of the importance of glucose as the basic coin of cellular energy exchange and the prevalence of diabetes, which manifests itself as renal disease along with other pathologies, we review the normal renal handling of glucose. The normal plasma glucose level is about 90 mg/dL (5 mmol/L). It rises transiently to well over 100 mg/dL during meals and can reach levels of over 1000 mg/dL (over 55 mmol/L) in severe diabetes. Normally, all the filtered glucose is reabsorbed in the proximal tubule. This involves removing glucose from the tubular lumen along with sodium via a sodium-dependent glucose symporter (SGLUT) across the apical membrane of proximal convoluted tubule epithelial cells, followed by its exit across the basolateral membrane into the interstitium via a GLUT uniporter. Unlike the case for sodium and many other solutes discussed later, the tight junctions do not manifest significant permeability to glucose. Therefore, as glucose is removed from the lumen and the luminal concentration falls, there is no back-leak. The transport of a solute with no back-leak depends only on the characteristics of the rate-limiting transporter, in this case the SGLUT symporter, and is a T_m-limited system.

Because glucose reabsorption is a T_m system, abnormally high filtered loads overwhelm the reabsorptive capacity (exceed the T_m; Figure 5–1). This occurs when plasma glucose rises above roughly 300 mg/dL. Again, this is a pathological situation but one that is relatively common. Assume that the glucose T_m is 375 mg/min (a typical value). The normal filtered load is well below this level. With a glomerular filtration

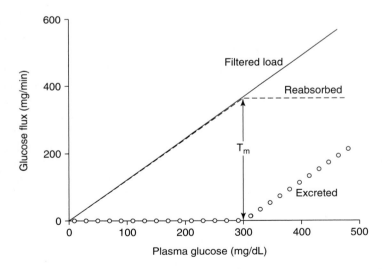

Figure 5–1. Glucose handling by the kidney. The solid line shows the filtered load. It is strictly proportional to the plasma concentration when the GFR is fixed at 125 mL/min. The reabsorption rate exactly matches the filtered load for loads less than the T_m of 375 mg/min. At all these loads, the excretion rate is zero. For filtered loads greater than the T_m, excretion becomes greater than zero and rises in equality with the difference between the filtered load and the T_m.

rate (GFR) of 125 mL/min (1.25 dL/min) and plasma glucose of 90 mg/dL, the filtered load is 1.25 dL/min × 90 mg/dL = 112.5 mg/min, much less than the T_m of 375 mg/min. When plasma glucose reaches 300 mg/dL, the filtered load is now 1.25 dL/min × 300 mg/dL = 375 mg/min. At this point, the proximal convoluted tubule fails to reabsorb all the filtered glucose, and a little glucose begins to spill into the urine. Further increases in plasma glucose above 300 mg/dL lead to progressively greater renal losses. We discuss the various reasons for diuresis (high urine volume) later, but one can appreciate that any glucose not reabsorbed is an osmole in the tubule that has consequences for water reabsorption.

PROTEINS AND PEPTIDES

Although we sometimes say the glomerular filtrate is protein free, it is not truly free of all protein. First, small and medium-size proteins (eg, angiotensin, insulin) are filtered in considerable quantities. Second, although the large plasma proteins are severely restricted from crossing the glomerular filtration barrier, a small amount does make it through. For albumin, the plasma protein of highest concentration in the blood, the concentration in the filtrate is normally about 10 mg/L, or roughly 0.02% of the plasma albumin concentration (50 g/L). Yet because of the huge volume of fluid filtered per day, the total filtered amount of protein is not negligible. However, the proximal tubule is capable of taking up filtered albumin and other proteins, and we treat this protein uptake separately here to emphasize its importance. We use the word *uptake* rather than *reabsorption* because the proteins, although they are transported intact out of the lumen into the epithelial cells, are degraded into their constituent amino acids before being transported into the cortical interstitium. Thus, the term *reabsorption* in the context of proteins and peptides, although widely used, is actually a misnomer.

The initial step for the uptake of larger proteins is endocytosis at the luminal membrane. This energy-requiring process is triggered by the binding of filtered protein molecules to specific receptors on the luminal membrane. Therefore, the rate of endocytosis is increased in proportion to the concentration of protein in the glomerular filtrate until a maximal rate of vesicle formation, and thus the T_m for protein uptake, is reached. The pinched-off intracellular vesicles resulting from endocytosis merge with lysosomes, whose enzymes degrade the protein to low-molecular-weight fragments, mainly individual amino acids. These end products then exit the cells across the basolateral membrane into the interstitial fluid, from which they gain entry to the peritubular capillaries.

To understand the potential problem associated with a failure to take up filtered protein, remember that

$$\text{Total filtered protein} = \text{GFR} \times \text{concentration of protein in filtrate}$$
$$= 180 \text{ L/day} \times 10 \text{ mg/L} = 1.8 \text{ g/day}$$

If none of this protein were removed from the lumen, the entire 1.8 g would be lost in the urine. In fact, almost all the filtered protein is taken up, so that the excretion of protein in the urine is normally only 100 mg/day. The endocytic mechanism by which protein is taken up is easily saturated, however, so any large increase in filtered protein resulting from increased glomerular permeability can cause the excretion of large quantities of protein.

Discussions of the renal handling of protein logically tend to focus on albumin because it is by far the most abundant plasma protein. There are, of course, many other plasma proteins, and it should be emphasized that many of these proteins, being smaller than albumin, are more easily filtered than albumin. For example, growth hormone (molecular weight, 22,000 kd) is approximately 60% filterable, and insulin is 100% filterable. The total mass of these filtered hormones is insignificant; however, because even tiny levels in the plasma have important signaling functions in the body, renal filtration becomes an important influence on levels in the blood. Relatively large fractions of these smaller plasma proteins are filtered and then degraded in tubular cells. Accordingly, the kidneys are major sites of catabolism of many plasma proteins, specifically including polypeptide hormones. Decreased rates of degradation occurring in renal disease may result in elevated plasma hormone concentrations.

Very small peptides, such as angiotensin II, are handled differently than larger proteins, although the end result is the same: the catabolism of the peptide and preservation of its amino acids. The very small peptides are completely filterable at the renal corpuscles and are then catabolized mainly into amino acids within the proximal tubular lumen by peptidases located on the luminal plasma membrane. The amino acids (as well as any di- and tripeptides generated by this process) are then reabsorbed by the same transporters that normally reabsorb filtered amino acids.

Finally, it should be noted that, in certain types of renal damage, proteins released from tubular cells rather than filtered at the renal corpuscles may appear in the urine and provide important diagnostic information.

ACTIVE PROXIMAL SECRETION OF ORGANIC ANIONS

The proximal tubule actively secretes a large number of different organic anions, both endogenously produced and foreign (see Table 5–1 for a partial listing). Many of the

Table 5–1. Some organic anions actively secreted by the proximal tubule

Endogenous substances	Drugs
Bile salts	Acetazolamide
Fatty acids	Chlorothiazide
Hippurates	Ethacrynate
Hydroxybenzoates	Furosemide
Oxalate	Penicillin
Prostaglandins	Probenecid
Urate	Saccharin
	Salicylates
	Sulfonamides

organic anions handled by this system are also filterable at the renal corpuscles, and so the amount secreted proximally adds to that which gains entry to the tubule via glomerular filtration. Others, however, are extensively bound to plasma proteins and undergo glomerular filtration only to a limited extent; accordingly, proximal tubular secretion constitutes the only significant mechanism for their excretion.

The active secretory pathway for organic anions in the proximal tubule in some sense is the reverse of reabsorption of organic solutes: There are active transporters for the anions at the basolateral membrane of tubular epithelial cells that are the rate-limiting step in overall transport. Transport out of the cell across the apical membrane into the lumen is via facilitated diffusion on a variety of uniporters or more specific sodium-dependent antiporters. Several different organic anion transporters (members of the OAT family of proteins) have been cloned. They are interesting in their similarity to amino acid transporters; they are specific for classes of organic anions (eg, OAT3 transports most tricarboxylic organic anions like citrate) but do not distinguish well among members of the class. Because the basolateral membrane of proximal convoluted tubule epithelial cells contains all of these different transporters, the proximal tubule has the capacity to secrete all the organic anions listed in Table 5–1 and many more. Like glucose, organic anions are not significantly permeable through tight junctions or membranes, so that their transport is also characterized by a tubular maximum. If the blood concentration of an organic anion is too high, it will not be efficiently removed from the blood by the kidneys (one aim of the dose regimen for prescribed drugs). The relatively nondiscriminating nature of this collection of transporters accounts for its ability to eliminate from the body so many drugs and other foreign environmental chemicals. In this regard, the liver's metabolic transformations are very important. In the liver, many foreign (and endogenous) substances are conjugated with either glucuronate or sulfate. The addition of these groups then renders the parent molecule far more water soluble. These 2 types of conjugates are actively transported by the organic-anion secretory pathway.

The most intensively studied organic anion secreted by this pathway is para-aminohippurate (PAH), the substance used for the measurement of effective renal plasma flow (see Chapter 3). PAH secretion involves a pair of antiporters, one at each membrane. At the basolateral membrane, PAH is taken up in exchange for the anion (base) form of a dicarboxylic acid. PAH is extruded into the lumen across the apical membrane via another antiporter.

As the plasma concentration of an anion secreted by this system increases, so does the rate of secretion (until the T_m for that substance is reached). This provides a mechanism for homeostatically regulating the endogenous organic anions handled by the system and for speeding the excretion of foreign organic anions.

PAH is typical, in yet another way, of many of the organic anions secreted proximally: It undergoes no significant additional transport anywhere along the nephron. In contrast, some of the other organic anions secreted by the proximal tubule can also undergo other forms of transport in both the proximal tubule and more distal segments. The most important of these is passive tubular reabsorption or secretion, which is described later.

Urate

Urate (the base form of uric acid) provides a fascinating example of the renal handling of organic anions that is particularly important for clinical medicine and is illustrative of renal pathology. An elevated plasma concentration of urate can cause gout; therefore, its removal from the blood is important. However, it is as though the kidney cannot make up its mind what to do with urate. Urate is not protein bound and so is freely filterable at the renal corpuscles. Almost all the filtered urate is reabsorbed early in the proximal tubule; however, further on in the proximal tubule, urate undergoes active tubular secretion. Then, in the straight portion, urate is once again reabsorbed. The total rate of tubular reabsorption is normally much greater than the rate of tubular secretion, and so the mass of urate excreted per unit time is only a small fraction of the mass filtered. We will not discuss the specific transport steps required to accomplish all of this, but most involve antiporters that exchange urate for another organic anion.

Although urate reabsorption is greater than secretion, the secretory process is homeostatically controlled to maintain relative constancy of plasma urate. In other words, if plasma urate begins to increase because of increased urate production, the active proximal secretion of urate is stimulated, thereby increasing urate excretion.

Given these mechanisms of renal urate handling, the reader should be able to deduce the 3 ways by which altered renal function can lead to decreased urate excretion and hence increased plasma urate, as in gout: (1) decreased filtration of urate secondary to decreased GFR, (2) excessive reabsorption of urate, and (3) diminished secretion of urate.

ACTIVE PROXIMAL SECRETION OF ORGANIC CATIONS

Proximal tubules possess several closely related transport systems for organic cations that are analogous to those for organic anions: Because of the large number of different transporters, a substantial amount of foreign and endogenous substances are transported (Table 5–2), the cations compete with one another for transport, and the transporters manifest a T_m limitation. Organic cations enter across the basolateral membrane via one of several uniporters, members of the OCT family (*organic cation transporter*), and exit into the lumen via an antiporter, which exchanges a proton for the organic cation.

The proximal secretion of organic cations, as for organic anions, is particularly critical for the excretion of those substances extensively bound to plasma proteins and not filterable at the renal corpuscle. However, again similar to organic anions, many of the organic cations secreted by the proximal tubules are not protein bound and, therefore, also undergo glomerular filtration and tubular secretion; creatinine is a good example.

Finally, and again analogous to organic anions, some organic cations are not only actively secreted by the proximal tubules but may also undergo other forms of tubular handling, mainly passive reabsorption or secretion.

pH DEPENDENCE OF PASSIVE REABSORPTION OR SECRETION

Many substances handled by the kidney are weak acids or bases. At a given pH, the total amount of each one is split between a neutral form and an ionized form. Many weak acids are neutral at low pH (acid form) and are dissociated into an anion and

Table 5–2. Some organic cations actively secreted by the proximal tubule

Endogenous substances	Drugs
Acetylcholine	Atropine
Choline	Isoproterenol
Creatinine	Cimetidine
Dopamine	Meperidine
Epinephrine	Morphine
Guanidine	Procaine
Histamine	Quinine
Serotonin	Tetraethyl ammonium
Norepinephrine	
Thiamine	

a proton at higher pH. The lower the pH, the more of the total there is in the neutral acid form, whereas the higher the pH, the greater is the fraction in the dissociated anionic form. In general, neutral forms of organic acids and bases are more permeable in lipid membranes than ionized forms, and the neutral forms can diffuse either into or out of the tubular lumen down the concentration gradient of the neutral form. In contrast, the ionized forms, once in the lumen, cannot diffuse; they are effectively trapped there. Imagine the case in which the tubular fluid becomes acidified relative to the plasma, which it does on a normal diet. For a weak acid in the tubular fluid, relatively more will be converted to the neutral free acid form and, therefore, become more permeable. This favors diffusion out of the lumen (reabsorption). Therefore, a highly acidic urine (low pH) tends to increase passive reabsorption of weak acids (and promote less excretion). For many weak *bases,* the pH dependence is just the opposite. At low pH they are protonated cations (trapped in the lumen), whereas at high pH they are converted to neutral free base. As the urine becomes acidified, more is converted to the impermeable charged form and is trapped in the lumen. Less is reabsorbed passively, and more is excreted.

Having said this, what difference does it make? Because so many medically useful drugs are weak organic acids and bases, all these factors have important clinical implications. For example, if one wishes to enhance the excretion of a drug that is a weak acid, one attempts to alkalinize the urine (because this traps the ionic form in the lumen). In contrast, acidification of the urine is desirable if one wishes to prevent excretion of the drug. Of course, exactly the opposite applies to weak organic bases. At any pH, increasing the urine flow increases the excretion of both weak acids and bases (Figure 5–2). Finally, excretion can be reduced by administering another drug that interferes with any active proximal secretory pathway for the drug.

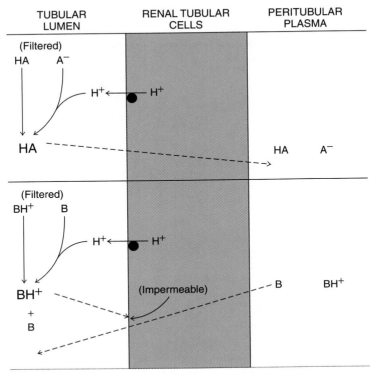

Figure 5–2. Acidification of the luminal fluid creates, by mass action, the gradients that drive net passive reabsorption of weak acids (*top*-dashedline) and net passive secretion of weak bases (*bottom*-dashedline). The source of the secreted hydrogen ions is discussed in Chapter 8.

UREA

Urea is a very special substance for the kidney.

It is both a waste substance that is eliminated (to maintain nitrogen balance) and a useful (necessary) factor in controlling water balance. Urea is produced continuously by the liver as an end product of protein metabolism. The production rate increases on a high-protein diet and decreases during starvation, but production never stops. The normal level in the blood is quite variable (3 mmol/L– 9 mmol/L),[1] reflecting variations in both protein intake and renal handling of urea. Over the long term (days to weeks), renal urea excretion must match hepatic production; otherwise, plasma levels would rise into the pathological range, producing a condition called *uremia*. On a shorter term basis (hours to days), urea excretion

[1] Plasma urea concentration is usually expressed as blood urea nitrogen (BUN) in units of milligrams per deciliter. Each molecule of urea contains 2 atoms of nitrogen, so 1 mmol of urea contains 2 mmol of nitrogen, with a combined weight of 28 mg. Thus, the normal levels of plasma urea are expressed as BUN values ranging from 8.4 mg/dL to 25.2 mg/dL. We use units of millimoles per liter because we can then directly convert to osmolality.

rate may not exactly match production rate because urea excretion is also regulated for purposes other than keeping a stable plasma level. As discussed in Chapter 6, urea is a key solute involved in regulating excretion of water. To summarize renal handling of urea, urea is freely filtered. About half is reabsorbed in the proximal tubule. An amount equal to that reabsorbed is then secreted back into the loop of Henle. Finally, about half is reabsorbed again in the medullary collecting duct. The net result is that about half the filtered load is excreted (Figure 5–3).

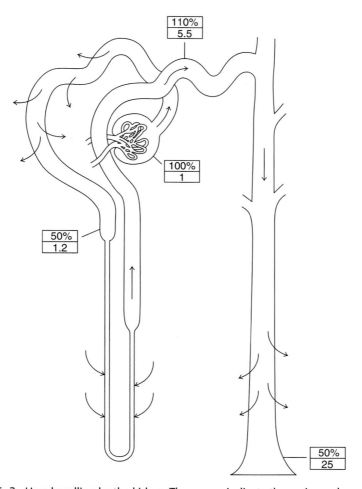

Figure 5–3. Urea handling by the kidney. The arrows indicate the regions where transport occurs and the direction of transport. The boxes show (in the top half) the percentage of the filtered load remaining in the tubule and, in the bottom half, the luminal concentration relative to the concentration in plasma. The numbers are subject to considerable variability, particularly for regions beyond the proximal tubule, because they are so dependent on hydration status.

As a molecule, urea is small (molecular weight, 60 d), is water soluble, and is freely filtered. Because of its highly polar nature, it does not permeate lipid bilayers, but a set of uniporters (the UT family) transport urea in various places in the kidney and in other sites within the body (particularly red blood cells). Because urea is freely filtered, the filtrate contains urea at a concentration identical to that in plasma. Let us assume a normal plasma level (5 mmol/L). Roughly half the filtered load is reabsorbed in the proximal tubule. This occurs primarily by the paracellular route. As water is reabsorbed (about two thirds of the filtered water is reabsorbed in the proximal tubule), solutes in the lumen that are not reabsorbed by the transcellular route become concentrated. Urea is prominent among these solutes. As urea becomes concentrated, it is driven passively through the leaky tight junctions. By the time the tubular fluid enters the loop of Henle, about half the filtered urea has been reabsorbed, and the urea concentration has increased to a little more than its value in the filtrate (because proportionally more water than urea was reabsorbed). At this point, the process becomes fairly complicated. First, conditions in the medulla depend highly on the individual's state of hydration. Second, there is a difference between superficial nephrons, with short loops of Henle that only penetrate the outer medulla, and juxtamedullary nephrons, with long loops of Henle that reach all the way down to the papilla. We simplify the issue and consider all nephrons together.

The interstitium of the medulla has a considerably higher urea concentration than plasma. The concentration increases from the outer to the inner medulla (part of the so-called medullary osmotic gradient), and its peak value in the inner medulla depends on hydration status and levels of the hormone antidiuretic hormone. We explain these variations in Chapter 6 in connection with regulation of water excretion. For now, we note that the medullary urea concentration is greater than in the tubular fluid entering the loop of Henle, so there is a concentration gradient favoring *secretion* into the lumen. The tight junctions in the loop of Henle are no longer permeable, but the epithelial membranes of the *thin* regions of the Henle loops express urea uniporters, members of the UT family. This permits secretion of urea. In fact, the urea secreted from the medullary interstitium into the thin regions of the loop of Henle replaces the urea previously reabsorbed in the proximal tubule. Thus, when tubular fluid enters the thick ascending limb, the amount in the lumen is at least as large as the filtered load. Because about 80% of the filtered water has now been reabsorbed, the luminal urea *concentration* is now several times greater than in the plasma. Beginning with the thick ascending limb and continuing all the way to the medullary collecting ducts (through the distal tubule and cortical collecting ducts), the luminal membrane urea permeability (and the tight junction permeability) is essentially zero. Therefore, a large amount (roughly the filtered load or more) of urea is still within the tubular lumen and flowing from the cortical into the medullary collecting ducts. The concentration is now much greater than in the plasma. Just how much greater depends on hydration status, because, as is discussed in Chapter 6, a variable fraction of the remaining water is reabsorbed in the cortical collecting ducts.

As tubular fluid flows in the collecting-duct system from cortex to medulla, additional water is reabsorbed. Thus, luminal urea concentration rises even more and can easily reach 50 times greater than in plasma. We indicated earlier that the urea concentration in the medullary interstitium is also greater than in plasma, but the luminal concentration is a little higher, so the gradient favors reabsorption in the inner medulla. Therefore, urea is reabsorbed a second time. In fact, this reabsorbed urea is the source of urea that is secreted into the loop of Henle. Finally, the result is that half the original amount of filtered urea passes into the final urine, an amount that, over the long term, must match hepatic production of urea if the body is to remain in balance for urea. These processes are summarized in Figure 5–3.

KEY CONCEPTS

The myriad array of organic solutes in the plasma is handled by the kidney; important metabolites are almost completely reabsorbed (saved), whereas waste products are, for the most part, excreted.

Most organic solutes are transported transcellularly by a large number of different saturable multiporters (T_m systems).

Normal filtered loads of glucose are completely reabsorbed by a sodium-glucose symporter that saturates at high filtered loads, leading to the appearance of glucose in the urine.

Urea is reabsorbed proximally and recycled between the collecting ducts and loop of Henle in the medulla.

STUDY QUESTIONS

5–1. *If 50% of a person's nephrons were destroyed, which of the following compounds would be likely to show increased blood concentration?*

   A. *Urea*

   B. *Creatinine*

   C. *Uric acid*

   D. *Most amino acids*

   E. *Glucose*

5–2. *The concentration of urea in urine is always much higher than the concentration in plasma. Is this because the overall tubular handling of urea is secretion?*

5–3. *If the concentration of protein in the glomerular filtrate was 0.005 g/100 mL and none was reabsorbed, how much protein would be excreted per day (assuming a normal GFR)?*

5–4. Suppose there is an excessively high filtered load of glucose, and only half is reabsorbed in the proximal tubule. How much of the remaining half now flowing into the loop of Henle is reabsorbed from this point on?

   A. None

   B. About half, leaving one quarter of the filtered load to be excreted

   C. Depends on hydration status

5–5. If you wished to increase your patient's excretion of quinine, a weak organic base, what change in urinary pH would you try to induce?

Basic Renal Processes for Sodium, Chloride, and Water

6

OBJECTIVES

The student understands the role of different tubular segments in the reabsorption of salt and water.

▶ *Lists approximate percentages of sodium reabsorbed in major tubular segments.*

▶ *Lists approximate percentages of water reabsorbed in major tubular segments.*

The student understands the role of the proximal tubule in reabsorbing the large filtered load of salt and water.

▶ *Defines the term iso-osmotic volume reabsorption.*

▶ *Describes proximal tubule sodium reabsorption, including the functions of the apical membrane sodium entry mechanisms and the basolateral sodium-potassium-adenosine triphosphatase.*

▶ *Explains why chloride reabsorption is coupled with sodium reabsorption, and lists the major pathways of proximal tubule chloride reabsorption.*

The student understands how the kidney can proliferate either a concentrated or dilute urine.

▶ *States the maximum and minimum values of urine osmolality.*

▶ *Defines osmotic diuresis and water diuresis.*

▶ *Explains why there is an obligatory water loss.*

▶ *Describes the handling of sodium by the descending and ascending limbs, distal tubule, and collecting-duct system.*

▶ *Describes the role of sodium-potassium-2 chloride symporters in the thick ascending limb.*

▶ *Describes the handling of water by descending and ascending limbs, distal tubule, and collecting-duct system.*

▶ *Describes the process of "separating salt from water" and how this permits excretion of either concentrated or dilute urine.*

▶ *Describes how antidiuretic hormone affects water reabsorption.*

▶ *Describes the characteristics of the medullary osmotic gradient.*

▶ *Explains the role of the thick ascending limb, urea recycling, and medullary blood flow in generating the medullary osmotic gradient.*

▶ *States why the medullary osmotic gradient is partially "washed out" during a water diuresis.*

OVERVIEW

Control of the renal excretion of sodium (Na), chloride (Cl), and water constitutes the most important mechanism for the regulation of the body content of these substances. Their excretory rates can vary over an extremely wide range. For example, some persons may ingest 20–25 g of sodium chloride/day, whereas a person on a low-salt diet may ingest only 0.05 g. The normal kidney can readily alter its excretion of salt over this range. Similarly, urinary water excretion can be varied physiologically from approximately 0.4 L/day to 25 L/day, depending on whether one is lost in the desert or participating in a beer-drinking contest.

Sodium, chloride, and water are all freely filterable at the renal corpuscle. They all undergo considerable tubular reabsorption, usually more than 99%, but normally no tubular secretion. Most renal ATP energy is used to accomplish this enormous reabsorptive task. The major tubular mechanisms for reabsorption of these substances can be summarized by 3 generalizations:

1. The reabsorption of sodium is mainly an active, transcellular process driven by sodium-potassium-adenosine triphosphatase (Na-K-ATPase).

2. The reabsorption of chloride is both passive (paracellular diffusion) and active (transcellular), but it is directly or indirectly coupled with the reabsorption of sodium, thus explaining why the reabsorption of the 2 ions is usually parallel. When describing the reabsorption of sodium, a parallel reabsorption of chloride is implied.

3. The reabsorption of water is by osmosis and is secondary to reabsorption of solutes, particularly sodium and substances whose reabsorption is dependent on sodium reabsorption (mostly chloride).

Sodium Reabsorption

Table 6–1 is a balance sheet for sodium chloride. Clearly, the major route of salt excretion from the body under normal circumstances is via the kidneys. The large amount excreted should not obscure the fact that nearly all the filtered sodium and chloride is reabsorbed. Table 6–2 summarizes the approximate quantitative contribution of each tubular segment to sodium reabsorption. In an individual with an average salt intake, the proximal tubule reabsorbs 65% of the filtered sodium, the thin and thick ascending limbs of Henle's loop 25%, and the distal convoluted tubule and

Table 6–1. Normal routes of sodium intake and loss

Route	Amount (g/day)
Intake	
Food	10.5
Output	
Sweat	0.25
Feces	0.25
Urine	10.00
Total output	10.50

Table 6–2. Comparison of sodium and water reabsorption along the tubule

Tubular segment	Percent of filtered load reabsorbed (%)	
	Sodium	Water
Proximal tubule	65	65
Descending thin limb of Henle's loop	—	10
Ascending thin limb and thick ascending limb of Henle's loop	25	—
Distal convoluted tubule	5	—
Collecting-duct system	4–5	5 (during water- loading) >24 (during dehydration)

collecting-duct system most of the remaining 10%, so that the final urine contains less than 1% of the total filtered sodium. As discussed in Chapter 7, reabsorption in several of these tubular sites is under physiological control by neural, hormonal, and paracrine inputs, so that the exact amount of sodium excreted is homeostatically regulated. Because so much sodium is filtered, even a small percentage change in reabsorption results in a relatively large change in excretion.

An absolutely crucial generalization is this: In all nephron segments, the essential event for active transcellular sodium reabsorption is the primary active transport of sodium from cell to interstitial fluid by the Na-K-ATPase pumps in the basolateral membrane. These pumps keep the intracellular sodium concentration lower than in the surrounding media. Because the inside of the cell is negatively charged with respect to the lumen, luminal sodium ions enter the cell passively, down their electrochemical gradient.

On examination of the luminal membrane depicted in Figure 6–1, note that there are various types of entry processes for sodium: Na-nutrient, Na-phosphate, or Na-sulfate symporters; Na-hydrogen (H) antiporters; and sodium channels. Quantitatively, the Na-H antiporters bring in the majority of the sodium (and serve as a major site for regulating sodium reabsorption in the proximal tubule). In other chapters, you will learn other roles of a particular segment besides reabsorption of sodium. For example, as discussed in Chapter 5, the proximal tubule reabsorbs nutrients, and the active step in this process is often by symport with sodium across the luminal membrane.

Another generalization that arises from the prior discussion is that you do not have to worry about any basolateral membrane transport processes for sodium except for the Na-K-ATPase pumps. (The function of the only other process shown in Figure 6–1, a Na-bicarbonate symporter in the proximal tubule and ascending thick limb of Henle's loop, serves to reabsorb bicarbonate, as is described in Chapter 9.)

Chloride Reabsorption

Because chloride reabsorption is dependent on sodium reabsorption, the tubular locations that reabsorb chloride and the percentages of filtered chloride reabsorbed by these segments are similar to those for sodium (see Table 6–1). When examining chloride reabsorption, it is helpful to keep in mind the absolute constraint of electroneutrality:

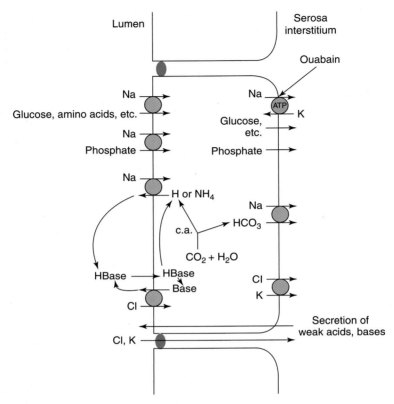

Figure 6–1. Major transport pathways in the proximal tubule. The entire proximal tubule is the major site for reabsorption of salt and water. The proximal convoluted tubule is the major site for reabsorption of glucose, amino acids, and other important organic substances and the major site for reabsorption of bicarbonate. The proximal straight tubule is the major site for secretion of organic acids and bases (including drugs). Because of the large amount of hydrogen ion transported (on the sodium-hydrogen antiporter) and the large amount of base equivalents transported (as part of chloride reabsorption), the presence of the enzyme carbonic anhydrase (both in the cell interior and on the luminal surface) is important for normal transport. Ammonium produced and secreted here is important for maintaining acid-base balance. ATP, adenosine triphosphate; c.a., carbonic anhydrase.

any finite volume of fluid reabsorbed must contain equal amounts of anion and cation equivalents. Let us do a "guesstimate" calculation. One liter of normal filtrate contains 140 mEq of sodium, and thus must contain about 140 mEq of anions, mainly chloride (110 mEq) and bicarbonate (24 mEq). (We say "about" because there are other cations [eg, potassium and calcium] and anions [eg, sulfate and phosphate] that must factor into the calculation to achieve an exact balance, but their contributions are much smaller than sodium, chloride, and bicarbonate.) If 65% of the filtered sodium is reabsorbed in the proximal tubule, $0.65 \times 140 = 91$ mEq of sodium in each liter of filtrate are reabsorbed. Therefore, about 91 mEq of some combination of chloride and bicarbonate must also be reabsorbed to accompany this sodium. As described in Chapter 9, about 90% of the filtered bicarbonate is reabsorbed in the proximal tubule ($0.9 \times 24 \approx 22$). This leaves $91 - 22 = 69$ mEq of chloride that must be reabsorbed in the proximal tubule. This is more than 60% of the filtered chloride and almost as much as the fractional reabsorption of sodium and water.

To understand active transcellular chloride reabsorption, it is necessary to recognize that the critical transport step for chloride is from lumen to cell. The chloride transport process in the luminal membrane must achieve a high enough intracellular chloride concentration to cause downhill chloride movement out of the cell across the basolateral membrane (of course, the movement of chloride across the basolateral membrane is also promoted by the negative potential within the cell). Thus, luminal membrane chloride transporters serve essentially the same function for chloride that the basolateral membrane Na-K-ATPase pumps do for sodium: They use energy to move chloride uphill from lumen to cell against its electrochemical gradient.

According to the luminal membrane depicted in Figure 6–1, the major routes are (1) paracellular absorption and (2) a complicated parallel set of Na-H and Cl-base antiporters (described later). These mechanisms are dependent on sodium movement across the membrane and are, therefore, linked to sodium reabsorption.

Water Reabsorption

With a large water load, the renal response is to produce a large-volume, very dilute (osmolality much lower than in blood plasma) urine. In contrast, during a state of dehydration, the urine volume is low and very concentrated (ie, the urine osmolality is much greater than in blood plasma). That the urine osmolality is so variable brings us to a crucial aspect of renal function. Terrestrial animals must be able to independently control excretion of salt and water because their ingestion and loss is not always linked (see Tables 6–1 and 6–3). To excrete water in excess of salt and vice versa (ie, produce a range of urine osmolalities), the kidneys must be able to separate the reabsorption of solute from the reabsorption of water to "separate salt from

Table 6–3. Normal routes of water gain and loss in adults

Route	ml/day
Intake	
Beverage	1200
Food	1000
Metabolically produced	350
Total	2550
Output	
Insensible loss (skin and lungs)	900
Sweat	50
In feces	100
Urine	1500
Total	2550

water." A dilute urine means that solute was reabsorbed in excess of water, essentially leaving the water behind in the tubule, whereas a concentrated urine means water was reabsorbed in excess of solute, leaving behind the solute. The latter case is tricky because, as we have emphasized, water always moves by osmosis from lower to higher osmolality regions. We later explain how this occurs.

A balance sheet for total body water is given in Table 6–3. These are average values, which are subject to considerable variation. The 2 sources of body water are metabolically produced water, resulting largely from the oxidation of carbohydrates, and ingested water, obtained from liquids and so-called solid food (eg, a rare steak is approximately 70% water). There are several sites from which water is always lost to the external environment: skin, lungs, gastrointestinal tract, and kidneys. Menstrual flow and, in lactating women, breast milk constitute 2 other potential sources of water loss in women.

The loss of water by evaporation from the cells of the skin and the lining of respiratory passageways is a continuous process, often referred to as *insensible loss* because people are unaware of its occurrence. Additional water evaporates from the skin during production of sweat. Fecal water loss is normally quite small but can be severe in diarrhea. Gastrointestinal loss can also be large in vomiting.

Water reabsorption always occurs in the proximal tubule (65% of the filtered water), descending thin limb of Henle's loop (10%), and collecting-duct system (where the fraction reabsorbed varies the most). A comparison of water and sodium reabsorption (see Table 6–2) reveals several important points. First, sodium and water reabsorption occur in the proximal tubule to the same extent. Second, both are also reabsorbed in Henle's loop. However, the part of the limbs involved in water reabsorption is different than for sodium reabsorption, but the fraction of sodium reabsorbed by the loop as a whole is always greater than that of water (ie, the loop overall is a site where salt is reabsorbed and excess water is left in the lumen of the nephron: "separating salt from water"). Third, sodium reabsorption, but not water reabsorption, occurs in the distal convoluted tubule. Fourth, both occur in the collecting-duct system. The percentages of sodium and water reabsorbed in the collecting-duct system vary enormously depending on a number of factors.

The movement of water down an osmotic gradient can occur by several means: simple net diffusion through the lipid bilayer, through aquaporins in plasma membranes of the tubular cells, and through the tight junctions between the cells. The amount of water that moves for a given osmotic gradient and its route depend on the water permeability of the different cellular component. The basolateral membranes of renal cells are quite permeable to water: The cytosolic osmolality is close to that of the surrounding interstitium. It is the *luminal* membrane and *tight junctions* where most of the variability lies. The segments of the renal tubule fall into 3 general categories with regard to water permeability: (1) The luminal membranes of the proximal tubule and descending thin limb of Henle's loop always have a very high water permeability; (2) the luminal membrane of the ascending limbs of Henle's loop (both thin and thick; recall from Chapter 1 that only long loops have ascending thin limbs) and the luminal membranes of distal convoluted tubule are always relatively water *impermeable,* as are the tight junctions; (3) the water permeability of the luminal membrane of the collecting-duct system is intrinsically low but can be regulated so that its water permeability increases substantially. These differences in water permeability account for the sites of water reabsorption as well as the large range of water reabsorptions given for the collecting-duct system in Table 6–2.

The ability of the kidneys to produce hyperosmotic urine is a major determinant of one's ability to survive without water. The human kidney can produce a maximal urinary concentration of 1400 mOsm/kg in extreme dehydration. This is almost 5 times the osmolality of plasma. The sum of the urea, sulfate, phosphate, other waste products, and a small number of nonwaste ions excreted each day normally averages approximately 600 mOsm/day. Therefore, the minimal volume of water[1] in which this mass of solute can be dissolved is roughly 600 mmol/1400 mOsm/L = 0.43 L/day.

This volume of urine is known as the obligatory water loss. It is not a strictly fixed volume but changes with different physiological states. For example, increased tissue catabolism, as during fasting or trauma, releases excess solute and so increases obligatory water loss.

The obligatory water loss contributes to dehydration when a person is deprived of water intake. For example, if we could produce urine with an osmolarity of 6000 mOsm/L, the obligatory water loss would only be 100 mL of water, and survival time would be greatly increased. A desert rodent, the kangaroo rat, does just that. This animal does not need to drink water because the water ingested in its food and produced by oxidation is sufficient to meet its needs.[2]

INDIVIDUAL TUBULAR SEGMENTS

Because we know that water reabsorption is driven by osmolality differences across the epithelium of water-permeable tubular segments, our major task in reviewing the individual tubular segments is to describe how these transtubular osmolality differences arise. We also explain how the kidneys can generate the osmolality differences by separating salt from water and form a hypo-osmotic or hyperosmotic urine.

The important principles to be understood regarding individual tubular segments are how the reabsorption of sodium, chloride, and water are related to one another and how the amount of reabsorption quantitatively varies from one segment to another.

Proximal Tubule

As shown in Figure 6–1, several luminal entry steps are involved in the active transcellular reabsorption of sodium in the proximal tubule. In the early portion (the proximal convoluted tubule), a large fraction of the filtered sodium enters the cell across the luminal membrane via antiport with protons. As described in Chapter 9, these protons, which are supplied by carbon dioxide and water, cause the secondary active reabsorption of filtered bicarbonate. Therefore, in the early proximal tubule, bicarbonate

---

[1] In this calculation, osmolarity is used as an approximation to osmolality to simplify the math.

[2] The obligatory solute excretion explains why a thirsty sailor cannot drink sea water, even if the urine osmolality is slightly greater than that of the sea water. To excrete all the salt in 1 L of sea water (to prevent a net gain of salt) plus the obligatory organic solutes produced by the body, the volume of urine would have to be much greater than 1 L.

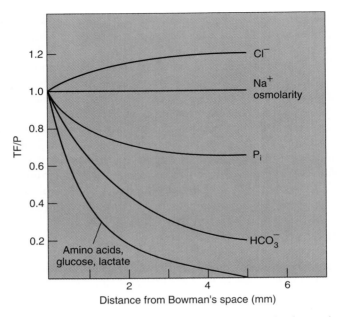

Distance from Bowman's space (mm)

Figure 6–2. Changes in tubular fluid composition along the proximal convoluted tubule. Values below 1.0 indicate that relatively more of the substance than water has been reabsorbed. Values above 1.0 indicate that relatively less of the substance than water has been reabsorbed. The concentrations of inorganic phosphate, bicarbonate, glucose, and lactate all rapidly decrease in the proximal tubule because these substances are actively reabsorbed much more rapidly than water. This is because these substances are preferentially reabsorbed with sodium in the early proximal tubule. In contrast, the concentration of chloride increases because chloride reabsorption lags behind sodium and, hence, water reabsorption in the early proximal tubule. TF, concentration of the substance in tubular fluid; P, its concentration in arterial plasma. (Modified from Rector FC, Am J Physiol 1983;249:F461; Maddox DA, Gennari JF, Am J Physiol 1987;252:F573.)

is a major anion reabsorbed with sodium, and luminal bicarbonate decreases markedly (Figure 6–2). Organic nutrients and phosphate are also absorbed with sodium, and their luminal concentrations decrease rapidly. We discuss sodium reabsorption in more detail later.

A major percentage of chloride reabsorption in the proximal tubule occurs via paracellular diffusion. The concentration of chloride in Bowman's capsule is, of course, essentially the same as in plasma (about 110 mEq/L). Along the early proximal tubule, however, the reabsorption of water, driven by reabsorption of sodium plus its cotransported solutes and bicarbonate, causes the chloride concentration in the tubular lumen to increase somewhat above that in the peritubular capillaries (see Figure 6–2). Then, as the fluid flows through the middle and late proximal tubule, this concentration gradient, maintained by continued water reabsorption, provides the driving force for paracellular chloride reabsorption by diffusion.

There is also an important component of active chloride transport from lumen to cell in the later proximal tubule. As illustrated in Figure 6–1, it uses parallel Na-H and Cl-base antiporters. Chloride transport into the cell is powered by the down-hill antiport of organic bases (including formate and oxalate), which are continuously generated in the cell by dissociation of their respective acids into a proton and the base. Simultaneously, the protons generated by the dissociation are actively transported into the lumen by Na-H antiporters. In the lumen, the protons and organic bases recombine to form the neutral form of the acid, and this nonpolar neutral acid then diffuses across the luminal membrane back into the cell, where the entire process is repeated. Thus, the overall achievement of the parallel Na-H and Cl-base antiporters is the same as though the Cl and Na were simply cotransported into the cell together. Importantly, the recycling of protons and base means that most of the protons are not acidifying the lumen but are simply combining with the base and moving back into the cells. It should also be recognized that everything is ultimately dependent on the basolateral membrane Na-K-ATPases to establish the gradient for sodium that powers the luminal Na-H antiporter.

Regarding water reabsorption, the proximal tubule, as mentioned, has a very high permeability to water. This means that very small differences in osmolality (1–2 mOsm/L at most) will suffice to drive the reabsorption of very large quantities of water, normally about 65% of the filtered water. This osmolality difference is created by the reabsorption of solute. The osmolality of the freshly filtered tubular fluid at the very beginning of the proximal tubule is, of course, essentially the same as that of plasma and interstitial fluid. Then, as solute is reabsorbed from the proximal tubule, the movement of this solute out of the lumen lowers luminal osmolality (ie, raises water concentration) compared with interstitial fluid. Simultaneously, it also tends to raise the interstitial fluid osmolality. This osmotic gradient from lumen to interstitial fluid causes osmosis of water from the lumen across the plasma membranes or tight junctions into the interstitial fluid. The Starling forces across the peritubular capillaries in the interstitium favor reabsorption, as explained in Chapter 4, and so the water and solutes then move into the peritubular capillaries and are returned to the general circulation.

The term *solute* was used to describe how reabsorption creates an osmolality difference between lumen and interstitial fluid. It should be clear by now, however, that we could just as well have referred simply to "sodium" because the reabsorption of virtually all solutes by the proximal tubule is dependent directly or indirectly on the reabsorption of sodium (Table 6–4). In other words, sodium and solutes whose reabsorption is coupled in one way or another with sodium reabsorption constitute the overwhelming majority of all solutes reabsorbed. Thus, the terms *sodium reabsorption* and *total solute reabsorption* are almost interchangeable when considering the proximal tubule.

Given the tremendous amount of sodium reabsorbed, how can the luminal sodium concentration and osmolality not progressively decrease along the proximal tubule? As shown in Figure 6–2, both remain almost equal to their values in plasma. Actually, the luminal values are slightly lower than the plasma values, but the difference is usually too small to detect. Remember that we are dealing here with concentrations of sodium and total solute (osmolality). Whereas 65% of the mass of filtered sodium and total

Table 6–4. Summary of mechanisms by which reabsorption of sodium drives reabsorption of other substances in the proximal tubule

Reabsorption of sodium
1 Creates transtubular osmolality difference, which favors reabsorption of water by osmosis; in turn, water reabsorption concentrates many luminal solutes (eg, chloride and urea), thereby favoring their reabsorption by diffusion.
2 Achieves reabsorption of many organic nutrients, phosphate, and sulfate by cotransport across the luminal membrane.
3 Achieves secretion of hydrogen ion by countertransport across the luminal membrane; these hydrogen ions are required for reabsorption of bicarbonate (as described in Chapter 9).
4 Achieves reabsorption of chloride by indirect cotransport across the luminal membrane (the parallel Na/H and Cl/base countertransporters).

solute has been reabsorbed by the end of the proximal tubule, so has almost the same percentage of filtered water. This is because the water permeability of the proximal tubule is so great that passive water reabsorption always keeps pace with total solute reabsorption. Therefore, the concentrations of sodium and total solute (osmolality), as opposed to their masses, remain virtually unchanged during fluid passage through the proximal tubule. This process, therefore, is called *iso-osmotic volume reabsorption.*

A good example of what happens when tight coupling between proximal sodium and water reabsorption is disrupted is the phenomenon known as *osmotic diuresis.* The term *diuresis* simply means increased urine flow, and *osmotic diuresis* denotes the situation in which the increased urine flow is due to an abnormally high amount in the glomerular filtrate of any substance that is reabsorbed incompletely or not at all by the proximal tubule. As water reabsorption begins in this segment, secondary to sodium reabsorption, the concentration of any unreabsorbed solute rises, and its osmotic presence retards the further reabsorption of water here (and downstream as well). Moreover, the failure of water to follow sodium causes the sodium concentration in the proximal tubular lumen to fall slightly below that in the interstitial fluid; this concentration difference, even though small, drives a net passive diffusion of sodium across the epithelium (mostly the tight junctions) back into the lumen (remember that the proximal tubule is a "leaky" epithelium and sodium transport is a gradient-limited system), resulting in more sodium than usual remaining in the lumen and passing on to the loop of Henle. Thus, osmotic diuretics inhibit the reabsorption of both water and sodium (as well as other ions). Osmotic diuresis can occur in persons with uncontrolled diabetes mellitus; the filtered load of glucose exceeds the tubular maximum (T_m) for this substance, and the unreabsorbed glucose then acts as an osmotic diuretic.

Henle's Loop

As stated earlier (see also Table 6–2), Henle's loop, taken as a whole, always reabsorbs proportionally more sodium and chloride (about 25% of the filtered loads) than water (10% of the filtered water). This is a key difference from the proximal tubule, which always reabsorbs water and sodium in essentially equal proportions.

Also as shown in Table 6–2, there is an anatomic separation of sodium chloride reabsorption and water reabsorption. The descending limb does not reabsorb sodium or chloride significantly, but it is quite permeable to water and reabsorbs it. In contrast, the *ascending* limbs (both thin and thick) reabsorb sodium and chloride but little water (because they are quite impermeable to water).

What are the mechanisms of sodium and chloride reabsorption by the ascending limbs? These are mainly passive in the thin ascending limb and active in the thick ascending limb. Water reabsorption in the descending limb (see later discussion) concentrates luminal sodium and creates a favorable gradient for passive sodium reabsorption. The epithelium of the thin *ascending* limb permits this gradient to drive reabsorption, probably by the paracellular route. As tubular fluid enters the thick ascending limb, the transport properties of the epithelium change again, and active processes become dominant. As shown in Figure 6–3, the major luminal entry step for sodium and chloride in this segment is via the Na-K-2Cl symporter (NKCC transporter). Na-K-2Cl symporter is the target for a major class of diuretics collectively known as the *loop diuretics,* which include the drugs furosemide (Lasix) and bumetinide. The luminal membrane of this segment also has a Na-H antiporter isoform, which, like the isoform in the proximal tubule, provides another mechanism for sodium movement into the cell.

The Na-K-2Cl symporter requires that equal amounts of potassium and sodium be transported. However, there is far less potassium in the lumen than sodium, and it seems that the lumen would be depleted of potassium long before very much sodium was reabsorbed. Interestingly, the luminal membrane has a large number of potassium channels that allow much of the potassium transported into the cell on the Na-K-2Cl symporter to leak back (ie, potassium recycles between the cytosol and lumen in order to be available for symport with sodium and chloride). Thus, under normal circumstances, luminal potassium does not limit sodium and chloride reabsorption through Na-K-2Cl symporters.

In addition to the active transcellular reabsorption of sodium, a large percentage (perhaps as much as 50%) of total sodium reabsorption in this segment occurs by paracellular diffusion. There is a high paracellular conductance for sodium in the thick ascending limb, and the luminal potential in this segment is positive, a significant driving force for cations. (We see in later chapters that this paracellular pathway also allows substantial reabsorption of potassium and calcium as well.) However, none of this would work without the continuous operation of the Na-K-ATPase in the basolateral membrane.

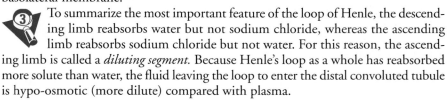 To summarize the most important feature of the loop of Henle, the descending limb reabsorbs water but not sodium chloride, whereas the ascending limb reabsorbs sodium chloride but not water. For this reason, the ascending limb is called a *diluting segment.* Because Henle's loop as a whole has reabsorbed more solute than water, the fluid leaving the loop to enter the distal convoluted tubule is hypo-osmotic (more dilute) compared with plasma.

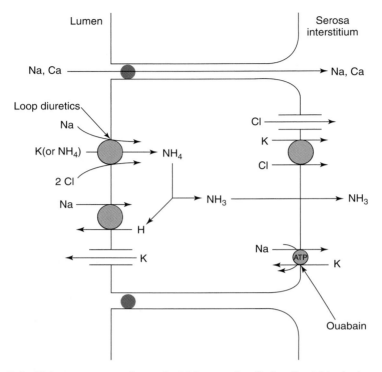

Figure 6–3. Major transport pathways in thick ascending limb cells within the loop of Henle. The major transporter in the thick ascending limb is the Na-K-2Cl symporter (NKCC), which is the target for inhibition by loop diuretics like furosemide and bumetanide. The apical membranes have a very low water permeability. In addition to NKCC, the cells contain an Na, H antiporter and potassium channels that recycle potassium from the cell interior to the lumen. Besides transcellular routes, some sodium and calcium also move paracellularly in response to the lumen positive potential. The thick ascending limb cells are the point in the nephron at which salt is separated from water so that water and salt excretion can be controlled independently. Defects in NKCC, the recycling potassium channel, and the basolateral chloride channel lead, respectively, to the 3 different types of Bartter's syndrome. Ammonium ion (produced in the proximal nephron) is reabsorbed here as part of normal acid-base balance. Besides the thick ascending limb cells, the thin descending limb cells apparently have no active transport with passive water reabsorption, with little or no NaCl reabsorption and passive entry (secretion) of urea into tubule. In the thin ascending limb in juxtamedullary nephrons, there is also apparently no active transport, but the apical membranes are relatively impermeable to water and urea, and NaCl reabsorption is passive. ATP, adenosine triphosphate.

Distal Convoluted Tubule

The major luminal entry step in the active reabsorption of sodium and chloride by the distal convoluted tubule is via the Na-Cl symporter (Figure 6–4), the characteristics of which differ significantly from the TAL Na-K-2Cl symporter and so are

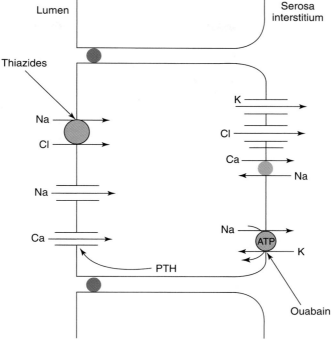

Figure 6–4. Major transport pathways in the distal convoluted tubule. The apical membrane contains the Na-Cl symporter (NCC), which is the target for inhibition by thiazide diuretics. There is also some sodium reabsorption via apical sodium channels (ENaCs). The DCT is also the major site for regulated reabsorption of Ca via apical Ca channels (under control of parathyroid hormone [PTH] and basolateral Na-Ca exchanger). A defect in NCC leads to Gitelman's syndrome. ATP, adenosine triphosphate.

sensitive to different drugs. In particular, the Na-Cl symporter is blocked by the thiazide diuretics, including hydrochlorthiazide. (Sodium channels, like those in the collecting tubule principal cells, also exist in the distal convoluted tubule.) Besides sodium and chloride reabsorption, distal convoluted tubule cells are a major site for the control of calcium homeostasis because they have apical calcium channels that are regulated by parathyroid hormone (see Chapter 10).

Collecting-Duct System

In the collecting ducts, there is a division of labor among several different cell types. Reabsorption of sodium and water is associated with principal cells (so called because they make up approximately 70% of the cells; Figure 6–5). Principal cells also play a major role in maintaining potassium homeostasis (see Chapter 8). Reabsorption of chloride can occur partially via paracellular pathways, but active reabsorption is also associated with another class of collecting duct cells, the intercalated cells (Figure 6–6).

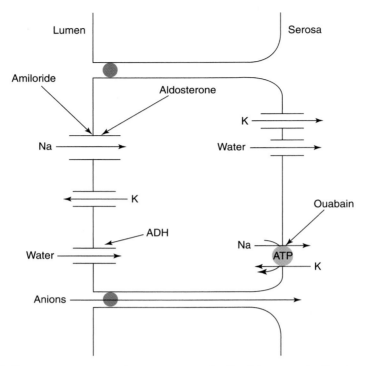

Figure 6–5. Major transport pathways in principal cells of the cortical collecting duct. The principal cells are the major cell type in the CCD. Sodium absorption is via apical sodium channels (ENaC). Activity of ENaC is controlled by the hormone aldosterone. Potassium secretion is via potassium channels and is driven by a concentration gradient and potential gradient. Water resorption is via aquaporin 2, the activity of which is controlled by the antidiuretic hormone (ADH). Some chloride reabsorption is passive via the paracellular pathway. ATP, adenosine triphosphate.

Different types of intercalated cells, besides mediating chloride reabsorption, also play a significant role in maintaining acid-base homeostasis (see Chapter 9).

The principal cells reabsorb sodium; the luminal entry step is via epithelial sodium channels. Regulation of this entry step is enormously important for whole-body physiology, and we expand on this topic in Chapter 7. Some sodium chloride reabsorption continues in the medullary collecting ducts, probably via some form of epithelial sodium channels.

 What about water reabsorption in tubular segments beyond the loop of Henle? The water permeability of the distal convoluted tubule is always very low and unchanging, similar to that of the ascending limbs of Henle's loop. Accordingly, as fluid flows through the distal convoluted tubule and sodium chloride reabsorption proceeds, virtually no water is reabsorbed. The result is that the already hypo-osmotic fluid entering the distal convoluted tubule from the thick ascending limb of Henle's loop becomes even more hypo-osmotic. Thus, the distal

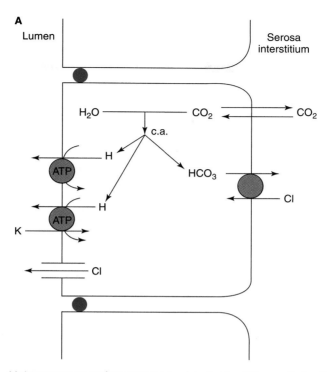

Figure 6–6. Major transport pathways in intercalated cells of the cortical collecting duct. The other major cell type in the cortical and medullary collecting duct is the intercalated cell. There are at least 2 types. **A,** A type A intercalated cell that is responsible for active secretion of acid as hydrogen ion via an H-ATPase and at least 2 isoforms of H-K-ATPase. The H-K-ATPase is also involved in potassium balance. Bicarbonate is returned to blood secondary to H$^+$ secretion (isohydric cycle). The acid secretion responds to aldosterone. **B,** A type B intercalated cell, which is responsible for active secretion of base as HCO$_3^-$ (isohydric cycle). H$^+$ is returned to blood secondary to bicarbonate secretion (isohydric cycle). The relative numbers of type A and type B cells depend on an individual's acid-base status. Type B cells are relatively rare in individuals whose diet contains any significant amount of animal protein. ATP, adenosine triphosphate.

convoluted tubule, like the ascending limbs of Henle's loop, functions as a diluting segment and further separates salt from water.

In contrast, the water permeability of the collecting-duct system—both the cortical and medullary portions—is subject to physiological control by antidiuretic hormone (ADH; see Figure 6–5). The inner medullary collecting duct has at least a finite water permeability even in the absence of ADH, but the outer medullary and cortical regions have a vanishingly low water permeability without ADH.

Depending on levels of ADH, therefore, water permeability for most of the collecting-duct system can be very low, very high, or everything in between. When water permeability is very low, the hypo-osmotic fluid entering the collecting-duct system

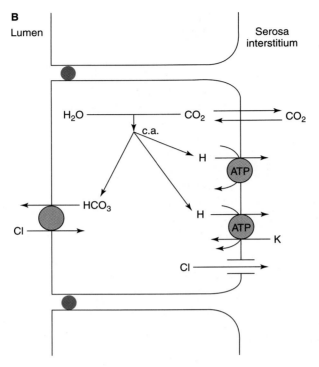

Figure 6–6. (Continued)

from the distal convoluted tubule remains hypo-osmotic as it flows along the ducts. When this fluid reaches the medullary portion of the collecting ducts, there is now a huge osmotic gradient favoring reabsorption, which occurs to some extent. That is, although there is little *cortical* water reabsorption without ADH (where most distal absorption normally occurs), there is still a finite medullary absorption because of the enormous osmotic gradient. However, because there is such a high tubular volume (ie, it was not reabsorbed in the cortex), most of the water entering the medullary collecting duct flows on to the ureter. The result is the excretion of a large volume of very hypo-osmotic (dilute) urine, or *water diuresis.*

In water diuresis, the last tubular segment to reabsorb large amounts of water is the descending limb of Henle's loop; in all later segments solute (mainly sodium chloride) reabsorption continues, but water reabsorption is minimal (although not zero in the inner medulla). Note that even when very little water reabsorption occurs beyond the loop of Henle, the reabsorption of sodium is not retarded to any great extent. Therefore, the intraluminal sodium concentration can be lowered almost to zero in these tubular segments, and the osmolality can approach 50 mOsm/kg. (This is possible because these tubular segments are "tight" epithelia, and there is very little back-leak of sodium from interstitium to tubular lumen despite the large electrochemical gradient favoring diffusion.)

What happens when the collecting-duct system's water permeability is very high instead of very low? As the hypo-osmotic fluid entering the collecting-duct system from the distal convoluted tubule flows through the cortical collecting ducts, water is rapidly reabsorbed. This is because of the large difference in osmolality between the hypo-osmotic luminal fluid and the iso-osmotic (285 mOsm/kg) interstitial fluid of the cortex. In essence, the cortical collecting duct is reabsorbing the large volume of water that did not accompany solute reabsorption in the ascending limbs of Henle's loop and distal convoluted tubule. In other words, the cortical collecting duct *reverses* the dilution carried out by the diluting segments. Once the osmolality of the luminal fluid approaches that of the interstitial fluid, the cortical collecting duct then behaves analogously to the proximal tubule, reabsorbing approximately equal amounts of solute (mainly sodium chloride) and water. The result is that the tubular fluid, which leaves the cortical collecting duct to enter the medullary collecting duct, is iso-osmotic compared with cortical plasma, and its volume is greatly reduced compared with the amount entering from the distal tubule.

In the medullary collecting duct (Figure 6–7), solute reabsorption continues but water reabsorption is proportionally even greater. In other words, the tubular fluid becomes more and more hyperosmotic and reduced in volume in its passage through the medullary collecting ducts because the interstitial fluid of the medulla is very hyperosmotic, for reasons discussed later.

How does ADH convert epithelial water permeability from very low to very high? An alternative name for ADH is vasopressin, because the hormone can constrict arterioles and thus increase arterial blood pressure, but ADH's major renal effect is antidiuresis (ie, "against a high urine volume"). In the absence of ADH, the water permeability of the cortical and outer medullary collecting duct is very low, and little if any water is reabsorbed from these segments, resulting in water diuresis. On the other hand, in the presence of high plasma concentrations of ADH, the water permeability of all regions of the collecting ducts is great, and only a small volume of maximally hyperosmotic urine is excreted. The tubular response to ADH is not all or none, however, but shows graded increases as the plasma concentration of ADH is increased over a certain range, thus permitting fine adjustments of collecting-duct water permeability and, hence, water reabsorption. (The control of ADH secretion is described in Chapter 7.) ADH acts in the collecting ducts on the principal cells, the same cells that reabsorb sodium (and, as is seen in Chapter 8, secrete potassium). The renal receptors for ADH (vasopressin type 2 receptors) are in the basolateral membrane of the principal cells and are different from the vascular receptors (vasopressin type 1). The binding of ADH by its receptors results in the activation of adenylate cyclase, which catalyzes the intracellular production of cyclic adenosine monophosphate. This second messenger then induces, by a sequence of events, the migration of intracellular vesicles to, and their fusion with, the luminal membrane. The vesicles contain an isoform of the water channel protein, aquaporin 2, through which water can move, so the luminal membrane becomes highly permeable to water. In the absence of ADH, the aquaporins are withdrawn from the luminal membrane by endocytosis. (As stated earlier, the water permeability of the basolateral membranes of renal epithelial cells is always high because of the constitutive presence of other aquaporin isoforms; thus, the permeability of the luminal membrane is rate limiting.)

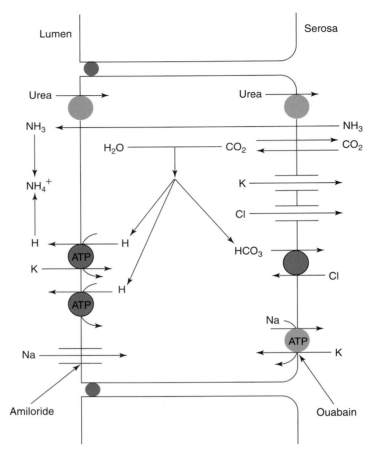

Figure 6–7. Major transport pathways in cells of the medullary collecting duct. The cells are responsible for hydrogen ion secretion and K reabsorption via H-ATPase and (H, K) -ATPase in the apical membrane (isohydric cycle). Ammonia secretion traps helps H⁺ in the lumen. Sodium reabsorption is via ENaC, and antidiuretic hormone (ADH) stimulates water reabsorption. There is also significant urea transport, some of which is constitutive and some stimulated by ADH. This schematic represents a summary of medullary transport processes. In reality, the transport processes are divided among several different cell types that are condensed here for simplicity. ATP, adenosine triphosphate.

URINARY CONCENTRATION: THE MEDULLARY OSMOTIC GRADIENT

The kidneys can produce urine that is hypo-osmotic, iso-osmotic, or hyperosmotic.

The production of a hypo-osmotic urine is, we hope by now, an understandable process: The tubules (particularly the thick ascending limb of Henle's loop) reabsorb relatively more solute than water, and the dilute fluid that remains in the lumen is excreted. The production of a hyperosmotic urine is also straightforward in that reabsorption of water from the lumen into a hyperosmotic interstitium concentrates that luminal fluid, leaving a concentrated urine to be excreted. The question is, how do the kidneys generate a hyperosmotic medullary interstitium? Not only is the medullary interstitium hyperosmotic, but there is a *gradient* of osmolality, increasing from a nearly iso-osmotic value at the corticomedullary border, to a maximum of greater than 1000 mOsm/kg at the papilla. (The maximum value depends on conditions; it is highest during periods of dehydration, and only about half of that during excess hydration.) Some aspects of how the kidneys generate a medullary osmotic gradient are still unclear. However, the essential points are clear, and it is these essential points on which we now focus.

The main components of the system that produces the medullary osmotic gradient are (1) active NaCl transport by the thick ascending limb from the nephron lumen into the interstitium, (2) the unusual arrangement of blood vessels in the medulla with descending components in close apposition to ascending components, and (3) the recycling of urea between the medullary collecting ducts and the deep portions of the loops of Henle (Figure 6–7 and 6–8). The actions of the thick ascending limb are the easiest to grasp. At the junction between the inner and outer medulla, the ascending limbs of all loops of Henle, whether long or short, turn into thick regions and remain thick all the way back until they reach the original Bowman's capsules from which they arose in the cortex. As they remove solute without water and dilute the luminal fluid, they are simultaneously putting solute without water into the surrounding interstitium (ie, they are tending to concentrate the interstitium). This action of the thick ascending limb is absolutely crucial. If transport in the thick ascending limb is inhibited (by loop diuretics that block the Na-K-2Cl symporter), the lumen is not diluted and the interstitium is not concentrated, and the urine becomes iso-osmotic. For those portions of the ascending thick limb in the cortex, the reabsorbed solute simply mixes with material reabsorbed by the nearby proximal convoluted tubules. Because the cortex contains abundant peritubular capillaries, the reabsorbed material immediately moves into the vasculature and returns to the general circulation. However, in the medulla, the blood flow is much lower, and it flows in the parallel arrangement described in Chapter 1. The low blood flow means that solute can accumulate in the medullary interstitium to produce an osmolality much greater than in the entering blood. (If there were no blood flow, solute could theoretically accumulate without limit, but medullary blood flow, although low, is finite). The low blood flow does not create the hyperosmolality but rather preserves it. Another major vascular factor is the physical arrangement of descending and ascending vasa recta running near each other in parallel. The specific permeability properties of the medullary vasculature and the exact osmotic content of the plasma in various regions are still uncertain, but, like other capillary beds, it is clear that solute and water can enter and leave the vasa recta. The plasma within them exchanges enough material with the interstitium so that the plasma osmolality at least approaches that of the surroundings; in other words, as plasma flows deep into the medulla, it becomes hyperosmotic. If blood vessels, which enter the medulla at the corticomedullary junction, were to leave the medulla at the papilla (ie, simply run straight through),

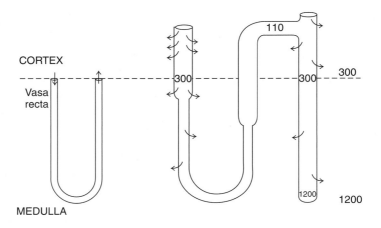

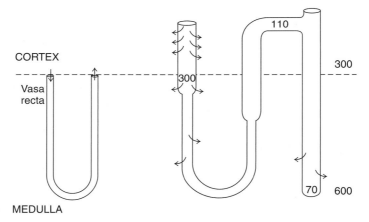

Figure 6–8. Renal water handling in states of maximum antidiuresis (**A**) and maximum diuresis (**B**). Numbers to the right indicate interstitial osmolarity, whereas those in the tubules indicate luminal osmolarity. Arrows indicate sites of water reabsorption. In both antidiuresis and diuresis, most (65%) of the filtered water is reabsorbed in the proximal tubule and another 10% in the descending loop of Henle. The relatively greater reabsorption of solute by the loop as a whole results in luminal fluid that is quite dilute in the distal tubule (110 mOsm). During antidiuresis, the actions of antidiuretic hormone permit further water reabsorption in the cortical and medullary collecting tubules, resulting in final fluid that is very hyperosmotic (1200 mOsm). During diuresis, no water reabsorption occurs in the cortical collecting tubule, but some occurs in the inner medullary collecting tubule. Continued solute reabsorption reduces solute content even more than water content, and the final urine is very dilute (70 mOsm). In the parallel vasa recta, there is considerable exchange of both solute and water, so that plasma osmolarity and solute concentration equilibrate with the surrounding interstitium. The vasa recta remove solute and water reabsorbed in the medulla. Because there is always some net volume reabsorption in the medulla even in states of diuresis, the vasa recta plasma flow out of the medulla always exceeds the plasma flow in.

they would remove a very hyperosmotic fluid and tend to wash out or remove the hyperosmolality of the interstitium. However, instead of leaving the medulla at the tip, the vasa recta change course and return to the corticomedullary junction. As the hyperosmotic plasma flows upward, it again tends to equilibrate with the surrounding interstitium, which is now decreasing in osmolality. Just as the plasma becomes more and more hyperosmotic on the way down, now it is becoming less hyperosmotic and approaching an iso-osmotic value as it flows upward. The flow of blood in parallel vessels in opposite directions and the ability of the vessels to at least partially equilibrate with the surrounding interstitium is called a *countercurrent exchange system* and is an important component of the medullary osmotic gradient. By itself, this countercurrent arrangement cannot generate the osmotic gradient, but it is crucial in preserving it.

The third element in the system is the recycling of urea. We described this recycling process in Chapter 5 and revisit it here. Urea (typical plasma concentration ≈ 5 mmol/L) is freely filtered, and about half is reabsorbed in the proximal tubule. Urea is secreted in the loop of Henle (thin regions), essentially restoring the amount of tubular urea back to the filtered load. From there to the inner medullary collecting ducts, little urea transport occurs, so whatever urea arrives at the thick ascending limb is still there at the start of the inner medullary collecting ducts. Because the vast majority of water has been reabsorbed by this point (by the cortical and outer medullary collecting ducts), the luminal urea *concentration* has risen up to 50 times its plasma value (500 mmol/L or more). In the inner medullary collecting ducts, some urea is reabsorbed via specialized urea uniporters (UT proteins; Figure 6–7). Because blood flow in this region is low, the reabsorbed urea raises the interstitial concentration close to that in the lumen (ie, 500 mmol/L or more depending on conditions). Typically, half the filtered load remains in the lumen and is excreted. If the interstitial urea concentration is 500 mmol/L, the interstitial osmolality must be at least 500 mOsm/kg, but, of course, it is much higher because there is a major osmotic contribution from sodium chloride. Usually urea constitutes about half the medullary osmolality and sodium chloride about half. As the medullary osmolality rises and falls with conditions (see later discussion), the concentrations of both components rise and fall. The key point for now is that, by recycling urea back into the interstitium, urea contributes greatly to the hyperosmolality of the medulla, allowing the kidneys to excrete a hyperosmotic urine. The importance of urea in generating the medullary osmotic gradient is emphasized in the case of low protein intake, which results in a greatly reduced metabolic production of urea. In this condition, the ability of the kidneys to produce a highly concentrated urine is compromised.

As already mentioned, the magnitude of the medullary osmotic gradient (actually the maximum osmolality found in the inner medulla) varies according to states of hydration. ADH, in addition to raising water permeability in the cortical and medullary collecting ducts, also raises urea permeability by stimulating a specific ADH-sensitive isoform of the urea uniporters but only in the inner medullary collecting ducts. Consider how this affects the medullary osmotic gradient. When a person is dehydrated, glomerular filtration rate (GFR) is somewhat low and levels of ADH are high. The extraction of water in the cortical collecting duct removes most

Table 6–5. Composition of medullary interstitial fluid and urine during the formation of a concentrated urine or a dilute urine

Interstitial fluid at tip of medulla (mOsm/L)	Urine (mOsm/L)
	Concentrated urine
Urea = 650	Urea = 700
Na$^+$ + Cl$^-$ = 750[a]	Nonurea solutes = 700 (Na$^+$, Cl$^-$, K$^+$, urate, creatinine, etc.)
	Dilute urine
Urea = 300	Urea = 30–60
Na$^+$ + Cl$^-$ = 350[a]	Nonurea solutes = 10–40 (Na$^+$, Cl$^-$, K$^+$, urate, creatinine, etc.)[b]

[a] Some other ions (eg, K$^+$) contribute to a small degree to this osmolarity.
[b] Depending on the sodium balance state, sodium in the urine can vary between undetectable to the majority of the osmolytes.

of the water from the lumen (and makes it iso-osmotic with the cortical interstitium). Then, as the remaining but greatly reduced, volume flows through the high osmolality medulla, further concentration occurs. The increased urea permeability signaled by ADH greatly assists in generating the medullary osmotic gradient by permitting the recycling of urea.

What happens in states of overhydration, as after a water-drinking (or other beverage) contest? Levels of ADH are now low. GFR is substantial. Only a small amount of the tubular fluid entering the cortical collecting ducts is reabsorbed there, and tubular urea does not become concentrated very much. A high volume of very dilute fluid with a modest urea concentration is delivered to the inner medullary collecting ducts. In contrast to the cortical and outer medullary collecting ducts, which are nearly water impermeable in the absence of ADH, the inner medullary collecting duct has a finite water permeability in the absence of ADH. Although this water permeability is not large, the osmotic driving force is huge, so substantial amounts of water are reabsorbed. (However, even more is not reabsorbed, and so urine volume is still very large.) Not much urea is reabsorbed; in fact, it may be secreted initially because the luminal urea concentration is lower than in the medullary interstitium. The result of the water reabsorption and the low (or absent) urea reabsorption is that the inner medulla is partially "washed out" (ie, the urea concentration and total osmolality of the medullary interstitium decrease over time). The osmolality falls to about half of its value (to 500–600 mOsm/kg) during maximum dehydration (Table 6–5). Thus, overhydration for several days before physical exertion (eg, a marathon run) with its associated loss of water as sweat may be counterproductive because the kidney will be unable to conserve water to the extent that it could if the medullary interstitium were normally concentrated.

Figure 6–9 summarizes the previously described changes in volume and osmolality of the tubular fluid as it flows along the nephron and emphasizes how, once fluid enters the collecting-duct system, the osmolality depends very much on levels of ADH.

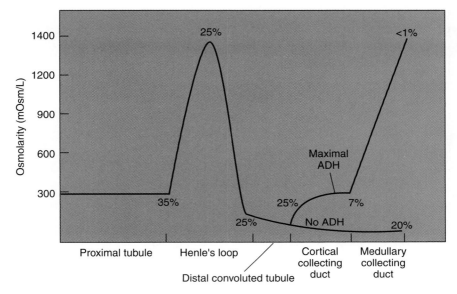

Figure 6–9. Osmolarity of the tubular fluid and the percentage of filtered water remaining at different sites along the tubule. The latter numbers, of course, are derived simply from the numbers given in Table 6–2 for the percentage of water reabsorbed by each tubular segment. ADH, antidiuretic hormone.

KEY CONCEPTS

 The reabsorption of most of the filtered water, anions, and osmotic content is linked to the active reabsorption of sodium.

 In all conditions, the vast majority of the filtered volume is reabsorbed iso-osmotically in the proximal tubule in a manner that is entirely dependent on active sodium reabsorption.

 The capacity to generate a variable-osmolality urine depends on "separating salt from water" in the diluting segments.

 Reabsorption of water remaining in the lumen beyond the loop of Henle is variable, depending on hydration status, allowing the kidneys to excrete either a high-volume dilute urine, a low-volume concentrated urine, or anything in between.

 Levels of ADH determine whether the hypo-osmotic fluid leaving the diluting segments is excreted largely as is or whether most of this fluid is subsequently reabsorbed.

The existence of the medullary osmotic gradient depends on (1) dilution by the thick ascending limb, (2) recycling of urea, and (3) low-volume countercurrent blood flow in the vasa recta.

 ## STUDY QUESTIONS

6–1. A man ingests 12 g of sodium/day. His nonrenal loss (gastrointestinal tract and sweat) is 0.4 g/day. In the steady state, what amount of sodium chloride is excreted daily in the urine?

6–2. Mannitol is a substance sometimes infused to reduce cerebral edema. It is handled by the kidneys similarly to inulin. What effect would a large mannitol infusion have on sodium excretion?

   A. No effect

   B. Increase sodium excretion

   C. Reduce sodium excretion

6–3. Complete inhibition of active sodium and chloride transport by the thick ascending limb of Henle's loop would virtually eliminate the ability to excrete a concentrated urine. True or false?

6–4. Increasing the passive permeability of the thick ascending limb of Henle's loop to sodium and chloride would reduce the maximal concentrating ability of the kidney. True or false?

6–5. Active reabsorption of sodium and chloride by the descending thin limb of Henle's loop is a component of the countercurrent multiplier system. True or false?

6–6. In conditions of maximum levels of ADH, there is net bulk flow of fluid from medullary interstitium into the vasa recta. True or false?

6–7. In conditions of minimum levels of ADH, there is net bulk flow of fluid from medullary interstitium into the vasa recta. True or false?

6–8. A drug is given that blocks all sodium channels and transporters in the luminal membrane all along the tubule but does not act on the Na-K-ATPase pumps in the basolateral membrane. What happens to sodium reabsorption?

Control of Sodium and Water Excretion: Regulation of Plasma Volume and Plasma Osmolality and Renal Control of Systemic Blood Pressure

7

OBJECTIVES

The student describes the renal regulation of extracellular fluid volume, total-body sodium balance, total-body water balance, and blood osmolality and their relationship to systemic blood pressure:

▶ *Describe the 3 temporal domains of blood pressure control and the major mechanisms associated with them.*

▶ *Describe the relationship between renin and angiotensin II.*

▶ *Describe the 3 detectors that can alter renin secretion.*

▶ *Define pressure natriuresis and diuresis.*

▶ *Define tubuloglomerular feedback and describe the mechanism for tubuloglomerular feedback and autoregulation of glomerular filtration rate.*

The student describes the renal regulation of total body sodium balance

▶ *State the formula relating filtration, reabsorption, and excretion of sodium.*

▶ *Describe the nature and locations of receptors ("sensors") in sodium-regulating reflexes.*

▶ *List the 6 factors that regulate sodium excretion.*

▶ *State the tissue origin of aldosterone, its renal sites of action, and its effect on sodium reabsorption.*

▶ *List the factors controlling aldosterone secretion and state which is normally most important.*

▶ *State the origin of atrial natriuretic peptides, the stimulus for their secretion, and their effect on sodium reabsorption and glomerular filtration rate.*

▶ *State the effect of antidiuretic hormone on sodium reabsorption.*

▶ *State all direct and indirect effects of catecholamines and angiotensin II on sodium reabsorption.*

▶ *Describe how intrarenal physical factors influence sodium reabsorption; state how changes in filtration fraction influence sodium reabsorption; predict the changes in physical factors that occur with changes in sodium or fluid balance and how they alter sodium and water reabsorption.*

▶ *Define glomerulotubular balance and describe its significance.*

▶ *Distinguish between primary and secondary hyperaldosteronism; describe the hormonal changes in each and the presence or absence of "escape."*

The student understands the renal regulation of total-body water balance and control of plasma osmolality:

▶ *Describe the origin of antidiuretic hormone and the 2 major reflex controls of its secretion; define diabetes insipidus; state the effect of antidiuretic hormone on arterioles.*

▶ *Distinguish between the reflex changes that occur when an individual has suffered iso-osmotic fluid loss because of diarrhea as opposed to a pure water loss (ie, solute-water loss as opposed to pure-water loss).*

▶ *Describe the control of thirst.*

▶ *Diagram in flow-sheet form the pathways by which sodium and water excretion are altered in response to sweating, diarrhea, hemorrhage, high-salt diet, and low-salt diet.*

As mentioned in Chapter 1, terrestrial animals, unlike their marine counterparts, have a unique problem. Normal function of virtually all organs and tissues requires that they be bathed in a medium of almost constant salt and water composition. This constancy must be maintained in the face of the ingestion of amounts of salt and water that are not only quite variable but often independent of one another (we rarely drink isotonic saline). Therefore, it is not surprising that there are independent mechanisms for the regulation of total body and plasma salt and water. However, there are also reasons for the coordinate regulation of salt and water leading to the excretion of isotonic fluid. In Chapters 4 and 6, we described the basic processes for renal handling of salt and water. In this chapter, we discuss the *regulation* of those processes. This is a Herculean task because we are facing what seems like a hopelessly complex jumble of interacting mechanisms. Our goal is to develop an orientation into ways of organizing one's thinking about the topic. We first provide a general overview and then examine the various elements more closely.

In regulating salt and water, the kidneys are actually regulating 4 quantities simultaneously: water balance, salt balance, osmolality, and blood pressure. The first 2 are seemingly straightforward: The kidneys regulate water excretion and salt excretion to balance their input. Osmolality is more complicated because it is not a substance that has an input and output; rather, it is the *ratio* of substances (solute and water). In essence, plasma osmolality is the ratio of the body sodium content (and its accompanying anions) to water content. Thus, a change in either water balance or sodium balance will change osmolality. Blood pressure is ultimately perhaps the most important regulated quantity. Blood pressure is crucial in salt and water balance because it plays an enormous role in generating the signals that alter water and sodium excretion by the kidneys.

REGULATION OF BLOOD PRESSURE

Regulation of blood pressure is a complex process that is not completely understood, but it involves a number of important concepts and components. First is the concept of a *set-point*, which is the value that blood pressure should be at any moment. The setpoint for blood pressure is like that for temperature on the thermostat in your house. Second, to regulate blood pressure near the setpoint requires *detectors* of blood pressure ("pressure gauges"), which assess the level of blood pressure at any moment. Third are *signals* generated in response to changes in blood pressure sensed by the detectors that communicate with the fourth component: *effectors,* which change what they do in response to the signals in order to raise or lower blood pressure and return it to the setpoint.

For simplification, we consider 3 contrasting temporal realms of blood pressure control: short-term, moment-to-moment control (seconds to minutes); intermediate-term control (minutes to hours); and long-term control (hours to days).

For each temporal domain, we examine how the setpoint is determined, the relevant detectors and the signals they generate, and how the signals impinge on the effectors to maintain the setpoint or balanced state. Short-term control involves the classic baroreceptor reflex that regulates cardiac performance and vascular resistances to compensate for changes in activity and posture. Intermediate-term control involves responses of renal sensors of blood pressure that lead to the production of chemical agents (renin and angiotensin II), which alter vascular resistances to correct blood pressure. Both of these control mechanisms alter blood pressure by changing the resistance of the vascular tree. Long-term control involves renal regulation of water and salt output to actually alter the volume of fluid within the vascular tree. The short-term mechanisms are able to influence the intermediate-term mechanisms; the intermediate-term mechanisms, in turn, are capable of initiating the long-term mechanisms; and the long-term mechanisms can provide feedback to determine the setpoint pressure around which the more rapid mechanisms operate. Despite this overlap between these systems in terms of mechanisms and interactions, it still helps to conceptualize them as separate but interacting processes.

Short-Term Regulation of Blood Pressure

Blood pressure is regulated around a setpoint controlled by a set of brainstem nuclei often called the *vasomotor center.*

There are 2 major types of detectors for the control of short-term blood pressure. The first are baroreceptors that mediate the classic baroreceptor reflex. These are afferent nerve cells (mechanoreceptors) with sensory endings located in the carotid arteries and arch of the aorta. They report arterial blood pressure to the vasomotor center via sensory neural pathways. The second are cardiopulmonary baroreceptors. These are also nerve cells, with sensory endings located in the cardiac atria and parts of the pulmonary vasculature. They are often called low-pressure baroreceptors because they assess pressures in regions of the vascular tree where pressures are lower than in the arteries. The cardiopulmonary baroreceptors serve as de facto blood volume detectors in the sense that pressures in the atria and pulmonary vessels rise when blood volume increases and fall when blood volume decreases. They, along with the arterial baroreceptors, send afferent neural information to the brainstem vasomotor center.

Based on the inputs from the arterial and cardiopulmonary baroreceptors, the vasomotor center sends regulatory signals to effector systems: the heart, blood vessels, and kidneys via the autonomic nervous system. Changes in the activity of the brainstem vasomotor center lead to changes in sympathetic signals that directly stimulate vaso-constriction or dilation of arterioles and veins, with consequent changes in periph-eral vascular resistance and central venous pressure (CVP). A decrease in blood pressure increases sympathetic activity, thereby increasing peripheral vascular resist-ance and CVP to produce a rapid return to close to normal blood pressure. In addi-tion to the effect on vascular resistance, sympathetic activity also alters heart rate and cardiac contractility to correct short-term changes in blood pressure. These fast effector mechanisms act immediately when pressure begins to change as a result of muscle activity or simple changes in posture.

The result of the signaling mechanisms is to stabilize arterial pressure at its setpoint, the mean arterial pressure, which for most people is slightly less than 100 mm Hg. The setpoint is not rigidly fixed; it varies during the day, depending on activity and levels of excitement, and decreases during sleep.[1] A complication lies in the fact that the value of the setpoint over the long term is actually determined by the kidneys (as discussed later). That is, the renal processing of salt and water ultimately deter-mines the average value of the setpoint for blood pressure of the brainstem vasomotor center. So long as the kidneys regulate salt and water excretion appropriately, the aver-age value of blood pressure over the course of a day will be normal. However, if renal excretion is inappropriate and remains so for several days, then the setpoint becomes reset to a new value.

As the name implies, short-term control of blood pressure through the barorecep-tor reflex and signals from the cardiopulmonary baroreceptors is a rapidly acting system that can respond to external perturbations in pressure on a time scale of a few seconds (1 or 2 heartbeats). Both of these types of pressure detectors work in concert to pro-duce sympathetic signals that maintain blood pressure nearly constant in the short term through vascular and cardiac effector responses. However, besides initiating rapid responses, changes in the sympathetic signals also have effects on the kidney that contribute to initiating the intermediate-term regulation of blood pressure.

Contribution of the Kidney to the Intermediate-Term Regulation of Blood Pressure

Although the kidney does not contribute in the short-term to control of blood pres-sure, the kidney is capable of strongly reinforcing the short-term vascular effects of the vasomotor center if a deviation in blood pressure is maintained longer than a few tens of seconds.

The major renal detectors involved in this intermediate-term regulation of blood pressure are pressure-sensitive cells within the kidney, often referred to as *intrarenal baroreceptors,* that sense renal afferent arteriolar pressure. Anatomically, these structures are not true baroreceptors but rather are specializations

---

[1] As an example of this variation, some patients experience "white coat hypertension," a phenomenon in which their blood pressure is normal while resting calmly at home but rises when a white-coated physician measures it in an office setting.

of the cells of the afferent arteriole: *granular cells* that form part of the *juxtaglomerular apparatus.* The intrarenal baroreceptors are not nerve cells and *do not* send signals to the brainstem vasomotor center. Rather, they act entirely within the kidney. Although granular cells acting as intrarenal baroreceptors do not send signals centrally, neural signals originating in the vasomotor center (generated in response to vascular baroreceptors) reach the granular cells via the renal sympathetic nerve. In response to changes in afferent arteriolar pressure *or* signals from the renal sympathetic nerves, the granular cells release the peptide hormone *renin.* When sympathetic stimulation increases because of a decrease in systemic blood pressure or there is a fall in renal arterial pressure, the granular cells secrete renin. Release of renin initiates a complicated series of biochemical events. Renin is a proteolytic enzyme that splits circulating angiotensinogen (a peptide produced in the liver) to form angiotensin I. Angiotensin-converting enzyme (ACE) in endothelial cells of capillaries (especially in the pulmonary bed but also the kidney) further cleaves angiotensin I to produce angiotensin II. Drugs that reduce the activity of this enzyme are popularly known as ACE inhibitors. Angiotensin II is a potent vasoconstrictor and increases total peripheral resistance and blood pressure. All of these events occur rapidly (but not as fast as the baroreceptor reflexes) in response to a decrease in blood pressure and represent a kidney-mediated correction for changes in blood pressure that reinforces the short-term changes caused by the vascular baroreceptors; however, angiotensin II-mediated vascular changes are initiated more slowly (tens of seconds or minutes) and are more persistent. The mechanisms involved in short-term and intermediate-term regulation of blood pressure are summarized in Figure 7–1.

Control of Renin Secretion

Although there are several steps in the production of angiotensin II, the primary determinant of the circulating levels of angiotensin II is the production and release of renin from granular cells. Therefore, understanding the control of renin secretion is critical to understanding renal control of blood pressure. Three primary detectors control renin secretion. Two have already been mentioned. The first are the vascular baroreceptors, which produce signals via the renal sympathetic nerves that stimulate granular cells: Activation of β_1-adrenergic receptors on the granular cells stimulates renin secretion via a cyclic adenosine monophosphate and protein kinase A-dependent process (Figures 7–2 and 7–3). Activity of renal sympathetic nerves also causes afferent arteriolar constriction and reduction in renal blood flow (RBF; Figure 7–4). The second detectors are the intrarenal baroreceptors. These receptors are granular cells that deform in response to changes in afferent arteriolar pressure; when the pressure falls, renin production increases (see Figures 7–2 and 7–3). Thus, granular cells act both as detectors (of renal arteriolar pressure) and effectors (releasing renin) in response to changes in pressure and sympathetic activity. The signals from the vasomotor system to the renin-producing granular cells ensures that there is tight coordination between the rapid activity of the baroreceptor reflex and the slower acting renin-angiotensin system; that is, the short-term regulation and the intermediate term regulation have at least one common set of detectors. Nonetheless, the intermediate-term regulation has a separate intrarenal pressure detector that can function in the absence

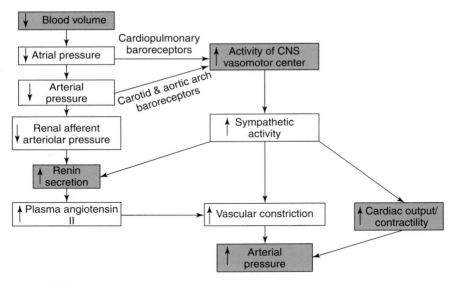

Figure 7–1. Short- and intermediate-term regulation of blood pressure. Abnormal blood pressure in either the arterial or venous side of the circulation is caused by a mismatch between the capacity of that segment of the vascular tree to hold blood and the actual volume within it. Short- and intermediate-term regulation of blood pressure generally involve altering both cardiac performance and relaxation or contraction of vascular smooth muscle. Both actions compensate for volume changes and, therefore, restore pressure. This figure demonstrates the sequence of events associated with a decrease in blood volume (eg, resulting from hemorrhage or severe diarrhea). The reduction in venous blood volume, where most of the blood resides, reduces filling of the heart, with a consequent reduction in stroke volume and arterial blood pressure. The reduction in arterial pressure and in volume in the venous system alters baroreceptors activity in several places, all of which activate the vasomotor center in the brainstem. Activation of the vasomotor center increases activity of the sympathetic nervous system. Increased sympathetic activity produces 2 major effects. The first is a direct effect on cardiac contractility and output and a constriction of the peripheral vasculature, both of which lead to a rapid short-term correction of blood pressure. The second is stimulation of granular cells of the afferent arteriole to release renin. In addition to the direct effect of sympathetic input on the granular cells, decreases in blood pressure activate intrarenal baroreceptors that also promote renin release. Circulating renin leads, through a series of steps, to an increase in circulating angiotensin II. Angiotensin II is a potent vasoconstrictor. Thus, the release of renin and production of angiotensin II strongly reinforces in an intermediate time frame the short-term effects of the baroreceptor reflex and sympathetic activation. CNS, central nervous system.

of renal innervation (eg, after a renal transplant). The third detector mechanism that regulates renin release is intrarenal and does not detect blood pressure directly. Rather, it measures the amount of sodium chloride that leaves the thick ascending limb, bathes the *macula densa* cells of the juxtaglomerular apparatus (see Figure 7–2), and is delivered to the distal convoluted tubule. This amount depends on both the rate of

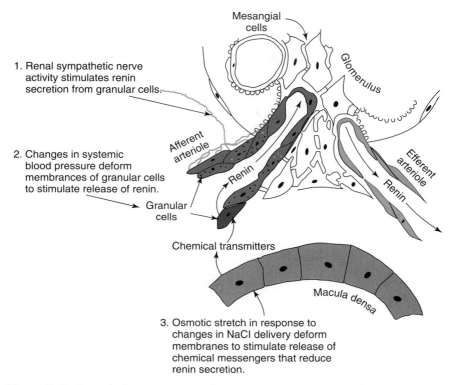

1. Renal sympathetic nerve activity stimulates renin secretion from granular cells.

2. Changes in systemic blood pressure deform membrances of granular cells to stimulate release of renin.

Afferent arteriole

Renin

Granular cells

Mesangial cells

Glomerulus

Efferent arteriole

Renin

Chemical transmitters

Macula densa

3. Osmotic stretch in response to changes in NaCl delivery deform membranes to stimulate release of chemical messengers that reduce renin secretion.

Figure 7–2. Control of renin secretion. There are 3 primary mechanisms by which renin secretion is regulated. First, when blood pressure falls, renal sympathetic nerve activity increases and activates β_1-adrenergic receptors on granular cells of the afferent arteriole to stimulate renin secretion. Second, the granular cells also act as "intrarenal baroreceptors." They respond to changes in pressure within the afferent arteriole, which, except in cases of renal artery stenosis, is a reflection of changes in systemic blood pressure. Deformation of the membranes of the granular cells alters renin secretion: When pressure falls, renin production increases. Third, macula densa cells in the thick ascending limb sense sodium chloride delivery by changing the uptake of salt, with subsequent osmotic swelling. Changes in cell volume lead to the release of chemical transmitters that alter renin secretion from the granular cells: When sodium chloride delivery increases, renin production decreases.

filtration and the rate of sodium reabsorption in all the nephron elements preceding the macula densa. Because filtration rate is regulated in part by sympathetic signals that vasoconstrict the afferent arteriole, the macula densa *sodium chloride load detector* integrates blood pressure and sympathetic activity with the reabsorptive capacity of the proximal nephron, loop of Henle, and thick ascending limb to regulate renin release. When sodium chloride delivery (a combination of concentration and flow rate) to the luminal surface of macula densa cells increases, renin production decreases (Figure 7–5). This is due to increased uptake of NaCl by the cells with subsequent osmotic swelling.

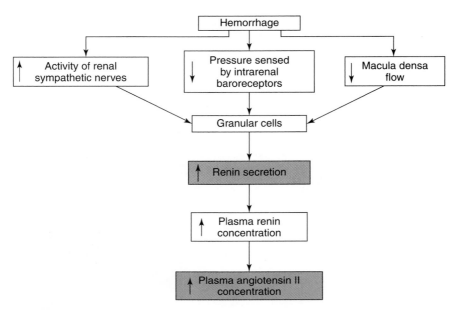

Figure 7–3. Schematic diagram of the control of renin secretion and the production of angiotensin II. Three primary mechanisms regulate renin secretion: (1) renal sympathetic nerve activity; (2) intrarenal baroreceptors (granular cell deformation); and (3) macula densa sodium chloride delivery sensors (osmotic swelling). All of these work in concert to promote renin release. Renin promotes the formation of angiotensin II, which produces strong vasoconstriction and helps to correct the decrease in blood pressure that resulted from the hemorrhage.

Osmotic swelling (Figure 7–6) causes release of transmitter agents (see later discussion) that inhibit renin release (see Figure 7–2). This load detector, therefore, provides one important way to couple the short-term (sympathetic activity) and intermediate-term (renin release and production of angiotensin II) regulation of blood pressure with the long-term regulation of blood pressure through control of sodium, chloride, and water excretion.

Besides these primary mechanisms, angiotensin II acts in a negative feedback manner to inhibit renin production by acting directly on granular cells (by interacting with AT1 receptors on granular cells to increase intracellular Ca concentration, which inhibits renin production).

CONTRIBUTION OF THE KIDNEY TO THE LONG-TERM REGULATION OF BLOOD PRESSURE

Despite the strength and efficacy of the vascular baroreceptor reflex and the potency of renin-induced angiotensin II in regulating vascular smooth muscle tone, these mechanisms are not the ultimate determinants of blood pressure in the long term. That is, the average value of blood pressure (or perhaps the average value of the setpoint

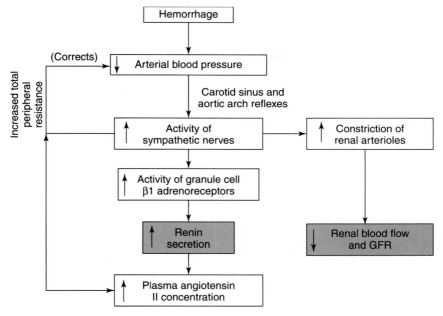

Figure 7–4. Sympathetic activity reduces renal blood flow. Besides the effect of symphathetic neurotransmitters on β_1-adrenergic receptors to stimulate renin release, they also stimulate α_1-adrenoreceptors (like those present on other vascular smooth muscle cells) to cause afferent arteriolar contraction and a reduction in renal blood flow. In the kidney, most of this reduction in blood flow is blunted by tubuloglomerular feedback (see Figure 7–8). GFR, glomerular filtration rate.

around which the baroreceptor reflex operates) is fixed not by the brainstem vaso-motor center but rather by the kidneys. Guyton and colleagues, in their classic experiments, surgically cut the neural pathways between the baroreceptors and the vasomotor center of anesthetized dogs. After recovery, the dogs' blood pressure varied widely from moment to moment, far more so than normal, but the mean value eventually returned to baseline. Various investigators ultimately showed that the kidneys are responsible for determining the setpoint for mean blood pressure.

How can the kidneys regulate blood pressure? Pressures in the vascular tree require an appropriate volume of blood (to fill both the highly elastic vascular tree and the chambers of the heart). Blood *pressure* in the long term depends on blood *volume*. Blood volume, in turn, depends on total extracellular fluid (ECF) volume (ie, the volume of blood plasma and fluid in the interstitial spaces of the tissues throughout the body). Fluid in the interstitial spaces acts as a buffer for plasma volume, protecting the vascular compartment from immediate changes associated with drinking, sweating, and so on. However, over time, sustained changes in ECF volume lead to parallel changes in arterial pressure. To keep arterial pressure normal (ie, keep a normal value for the setpoint around which the baroreceptor reflex operates), the ECF volume must be kept normal. This is the job of the kidneys.

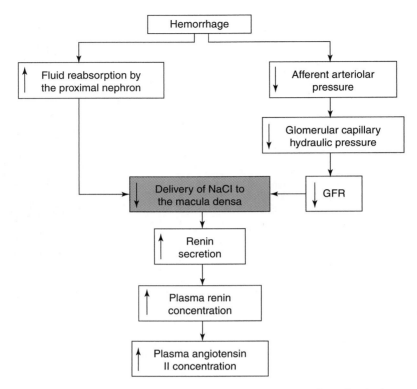

Figure 7–5. The macula densa NaCl load sensor. Macula densa cells in the thick ascending limb sense sodium chloride delivery by changing the uptake of salt with subsequent osmotic swelling (see Figure 7–6). Changes in cell volume lead to the release of chemical transmitters that alter renin secretion from the granular cells: When sodium chloride delivery increases, renin production decreases. GFR, glomerular filtration rate.

 Note: In many ways, regulating the ECF volume to a level appropriate for the vascular system (and consequently determining the set point for mean blood pressure) is the most important function of the kidneys!

It is worth emphasizing the time lag between volume changes and pressure changes. For example, increasing volume by ingesting a large amount of liquid or decreasing volume by sweating during a tennis match on a hot day does not immediately cause changes in blood pressure. This is because tendencies to change pressure are buffered by the classic baroreceptor reflex, and the kidneys change their output of salt and water to match the input. However, if the kidneys do not match their output to input, and changes in ECF volume are sustained, then pressure gradually creeps toward a new elevated or depressed value. In the face of sustained changes in volume, the baroreceptor reflex cannot forever keep pressure normal. We are unaware of the kidneys' role in the control of blood pressure because the baroreceptor reflex is very effective on a short-term

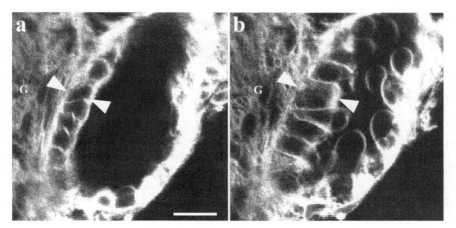

Figure 7–6. Responses of macula densa cells to changes in delivery of NaCl load. The macula densa cells (arrowheads) are in close apposition to the glomerulus (G). Macula densa cells swell in response to increasing tubular NaCl concentration from 25 (total osmolality = 210 mOsm/kg H_2O) on the left to 135 mmol (total osmolality = 300 mOsm/kg H_2O). Bar = 10 μm. From Peti-Peterdi J et al, Am J Physiol Renal Physiol 2002;283;F197. Used with permission.)

basis in buffering changes and because healthy kidneys do such a good job of adjusting their volume output in the face of changes in input.

Sodium and Water Connection

As mentioned, blood volume over time determines blood pressure. The relationship between blood volume and total body water may appear obvious, but the relationship between total body sodium content and blood volume may not. However, as discussed in Chapter 4, there is a simple relation between volume of a compartment (essentially the amount of water) and its osmolarity: osmolarity = total osmoles/volume.[2] In other words, volume = total osmoles/osmolarity. Therefore, the ECF volume is determined by the total osmotic content and osmolarity. If the body regulates the total osmotic content of the ECF and regulates its osmolarity, it has accomplished the task of regulating its volume. This is precisely what the kidneys do. They regulate ECF osmolarity and total osmotic content.

Recall that more than 90% of the ECF osmotic content is accounted for by sodium and the equal number of anions that must accompany it. To a first approximation, total ECF osmotic content = sodium content × 2. The other 10% of the ECF solute is accounted for by substances such as potassium, glucose, urea, and so on. The regulation of solutes other than sodium occurs for purposes unrelated to control of ECF

---

[2] Here again, we use osmolarity for simplicity, recognizing that *osmolality* is actually the quantity that governs osmotic flow.

osmolality, so that regulation of osmotic content amounts to regulation of sodium content.

In simple terms, long-term regulation of blood pressure involves long-term control of body sodium content. If the body controls sodium content and plasma molarity (the water content containing the sodium), it controls volume. If it controls volume, it controls pressure.

How do the kidneys receive information about sodium content to which they can respond? Surprisingly, in detecting total body sodium, the primary variable that the kidney monitors is not total body sodium or plasma sodium but rather systemic blood pressure (sensed by all of the vascular and renal baroreceptor-sensing mechanisms described previously). Pressure changes at any of these sites is interpreted as a change in total body sodium because, except for pathophysiological circumstances, blood pressure, blood volume, and total body sodium march in lockstep. The most important detectors of vascular pressure that affect renal function are the kidneys themselves!

Pressure Natriuresis and Diuresis

The intrarenal baroreceptors respond to pressures in the renal vasculature. Elevated pressure in the renal artery is interpreted by the kidney as both excess plasma sodium and excess plasma volume. Such an increase in renal artery pressure, independent of any signals external to the kidney, increases the excretion of sodium and water. These increases in excretion are called *pressure natriuresis* (an increased sodium content of the urine as a result of elevated blood pressure) and increases excretion of water, or *pressure diuresis* (an increased volume of urine). This makes eminent sense. If the body accumulates sodium, blood volume increases, and blood pressure begins to creep up over time, then pressure natriuresis accelerates sodium excretion and pressure diuresis increases water excretion. The kidney, in effect, excretes isotonic urine to reduce blood volume (and blood pressure). A significant part of this mechanism lies in reducing sodium absorption in the proximal tubule. Recall that much of the sodium entry into the epithelial cells is via Na-H antiporters. In response to elevated renal artery pressure, the number of these transporters in the apical membrane is reduced, along with a concomitant reduction in activity of the basolateral Na-K-ATPase. The result is less sodium absorption and more presentation of sodium to the loop of Henle. The activity of the proximal Na-H exchange and Na-K-ATPase appears to depend on renal levels of angiotensin II and sympathetic transmitter agents. If peritubular levels of angiotensin II are maintained constant regardless of increases in systemic blood pressure (when angiotensin II would normally decrease), pressure natriuresis and diuresis are strongly blunted or even eliminated. The effect of maintaining constant sympathetic transmitters is similar but not so pronounced. Thus, the same agents that directly effect the vasculature to correct blood pressure also affect tubular reabsorption to correct ECF volume.

A key feature of pressure natriuresis and diuresis is that the degree of salt and water excretion for a given rise in pressure varies with the volume status of the body. If the ECF volume is normal or high and pressure in the renal artery rises, pressure natriuresis and diuresis are very effective in increasing excretion of sodium and water and reducing blood volume. On the other hand, if ECF volume is low and renal artery pressure rises, there is much less salt and water loss. It appears that the volume status of the body acts as a gain control on pressure natriuresis and diuresis.[3] There is potent pressure natriuresis and diuresis when ECF volume is high and much less pressure natriuresis and diuresis when ECF volume is depleted. Thus, pressure diuresis is a proximal nephron mechanism that is very important for reducing ECF volume when blood pressure is too high. It does this by reducing isotonic reabsorption of salt and water from the proximal convoluted and straight tubule. However, although pressure natriuresis and diuresis are effective at controlling ECF volume and, therefore, blood pressure, it is not particularly useful for *independently* controlling salt or water excretion because pressure diuresis and natriuresis almost always go hand in hand. Independent control of total body sodium or water content requires additional specific hormonal mechanisms described later. Nonetheless, the characteristics of pressure natriuresis and diuresis again emphasize the key role of the kidneys in maintaining an ECF volume that is appropriate for the vascular system (Figure 7–7).

Control of Glomerular Filtration Rate

Because sodium excretion represents the difference between filtration and reabsorption, it is not surprising that regulation of glomerular filtration rate (GFR) plays a role in the regulation of sodium excretion. However, as in the case of pressure natriuresis, a change in the amount of sodium filtered resulting from a change in GFR is also accompanied by a change in the amount of water filtered. Therefore, any change in GFR also represents a mechanism for altering ECF volume rather than independently regulating salt and water.

The reflex control of GFR is mediated mainly by changing the resistance of the afferent and efferent arteriolar resistance. The changes in resistance are produced by changes in renal sympathetic nerve activity and circulating levels of angiotensin II. (As described later, antidiuretic hormone [ADH] and *natriuretic peptide* hormones can also play significant physiological roles under certain circumstances.) These reflexes and the detailed mechanisms by which they lower GFR have already been described in Chapter 2 (see Figures 2–6 to 2–10).

For further review, Figure 7–7 provides another example of how the sympathetic nerves and angiotensin II are reflexively increased by a decrease in plasma volume and produce a small decrease in GFR. By these reflexes, the amount of sodium and water filtered, and hence the amount excreted, is reduced, and further loss from the body is minimized.

Conversely, renal sympathetic nerve activity and renin secretion are reflexively decreased when plasma volume is increased physiologically. However, in a person ingesting the usual American diet, which contains relatively large amounts of sodium, sympathetic activity is usually so low that a further decrease has little or no effect on GFR (or RBF).

---

[3] This is one of the unknowns of renal function. Although mechanical stretch of the afferent arterioles can transduce blood pressure into cellular responses, it is not clear how the kidney senses volume status independently of signals generated via baroreceptors outside the kidneys.

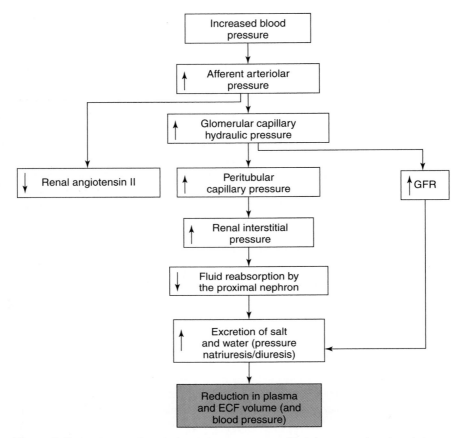

Figure 7–7. Response of the kidneys to an increase in blood pressure (natriuresis/diuresis). Part of the intermediate-term response to increases in blood pressure is to reduce blood volume (in an attempt to match blood volume with the capacity of the vascular tree). There are several mechanisms for this response. By far, the most important is a reduction in proximal tubular sodium reabsorption because of a reduction in the number of functional transporters (Na-H antiporters) in the apical membrane of the proximal tubule epithelial cells. The reduction is probably in response to reduced levels of angiotensin II. There is also an increase (usually small) in glomerular filtration rate (GFR) and an increase in peritubular hydrostatic pressure and renal interstitial pressure that favor reduced absorption of salt and water in the cortex (particularly from the proximal nephron). ECF, extracellular fluid.

Tubuloglomerular Feedback and Autoregulation Revisited

Pressure natriuresis and diuresis are extremely effective mechanisms for controlling blood volume. Changes in GFR mediated by changes in afferent arteriolar resistance add further control. Although this change in afferent resistance has the effect of altering GFR in a manner necessary to correct blood volume, it has the additional consequence of altering RBF and pressure in the glomerular capillaries. Both of these effects may have deleterious consequences. Substantial reductions in RBF will severely compromise already oxygen-poor regions of the kidney like the medulla. Substantial increases in glomerular capillary pressures are likely to damage the glomeruli. In addition, the ability of the kidney to correct total body electrolyte and water imbalances depends on keeping tubular flow (ie, GFR) within a certain limited range. Therefore, the kidney has specific mechanisms for blunting responses that would otherwise lead to large changes in GFR (*autoregulation*) or RBF (*tubuloglomerular feedback*). The mechanism for autoregulation of GFR involves local production of *prostaglandins*. Intrarenal (autoregulatory) prostaglandin production opposes the actions of angiotensin II on the kidneys; that is, prostaglandins lead to vasodilation of arterioles and relaxation of mesangial cells (Figure 7–8). Increased local (intrarenal) angiotensin II concentrations associated with renin release and increased sympathetic input stimulate production of prostaglandins. The vasodilatory effect of prostaglandins dampens the effect of angiotensin II and sympathetic input on renal arterioles (intrarenal effect only; ie, prostaglandin production opposes the constrictive effects of angiotensin II and norepinephrine on afferent arteriolar smooth muscle and mesangial cells to maintain RBF and GFR despite systemic vasoconstriction.

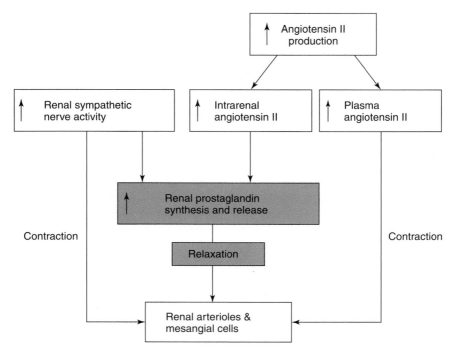

Figure 7–8. Prostaglandins mediate autoregulatory responses. Production of prostaglandins (mostly PGE$_2$) near the glomerulus relaxes the afferent arteriole and thus counteracts the contractile effects of renal sympathetic nerve activation and angiotensin II.

Tubuloglomerular feedback, alternatively, is associated with the macula densa sodium chloride load detector. The macula densa cells have Na-K-2Cl symporters that can avidly take up Na, Cl, and K and cause the cells to swell dramatically when GFR (NaCl delivery) is high (see Figure 7–6). The increased Na and Cl in the lumen of the thick ascending limb stimulates the Na-H antiporter and depolarizes the cells (as in thick ascending limb cells, the K recycles via K channels. This depolarization leads to Ca entry across the basolateral membrane. The rise in Ca leads to the release of ATP from the basolateral surface of the cells in close proximity to the glomerular mesangial cells. This ATP stimulates purinergic P2 receptors on the mesangial cells and afferent arteriolar smooth muscle cells. P2 receptor stimulation increases Ca in these cells and promotes contraction. In addition (as described previously), the increased Ca in the afferent arteriolar cells reduces renin secretion. The ATP may also be metabolized to adenosine, which can stimulate adenosine receptors that produce the same result as the P2 receptors (in contrast to the vasodilatory actions of adenosine in most other tissues).[4] Contraction of mesangial cells decreases the effective filtration area, which decreases GFR. Contraction of the afferent arteriolar smooth muscle cells increases afferent resistance and decreases RBF and GFR. As a relatively minor contribution, the increase in intracellular Ca of the granular cells inhibits their production of intrarenal renin, thus reducing local production of angiotensin II and of prostaglandins, which would normally counteract the vasoconstrictive effects of the purinergic agonists. Another mediator—nitric oxide (NO)—is not a factor in initiating tubuloglomerular feedback but does appear to play a secondary role to sustain the tubuloglomerular feedback once it has been initiated. The net effect of tubuloglomerular feedback is that the pressure natriuretic and diuretic responses are blunted (but not eliminated), and other aspects of renal tubular function are uncompromised (Figures 7–9 and 7–10).

Peritubular-Capillary Starling Factors and the Role of Renal Interstitial Hydraulic Pressure

A rise in either peritubular capillary pressure or interstitial pressure reduces net reabsorption. Why? First, an increased interstitial pressure causes back-leak of reabsorbed fluid from the interstitial space across the tight junctions into the tubule. Thus, this effect does not alter the cellular transport mechanisms for sodium and water but rather reduces the net reabsorption achieved by these mechanisms, particularly in the "leaky" proximal tubule. In effect, if the interstitium gets "too full," it is difficult to transport more fluid into it. Second, an increase in peritubular-capillary hydraulic pressure (P_{PC}) reduces the force favoring movement of interstitial fluid into the capillaries, which causes fluid to accumulate in the interstitium, thereby raising interstitial pressure. A decrease in peritubular-capillary oncotic pressure (π_{PC}) does the same thing. Of course, the new question is: What causes changes in P_{PC} and π_{PC}? We already know the answers to this question from Chapter 2: P_{PC} is set by (1) arterial

---

[4] The actions of adenosine in a given cell depend on the type of purinergic receptor and the signaling pathway initiated on binding of adenosine, similar to the situation with adrenergic receptors, in which an array of receptor types permits a variety of responses to any given agonist.

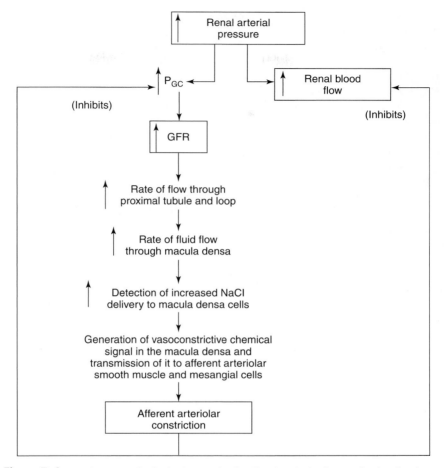

Figure 7–9. Mechanism of tubuloglomerular feedback. Tubuloglomerular feedback acts to prevent changes in renal artery pressure from causing extreme changes in sodium delivery to the macula densa. This mechanism acts in the opposite direction to the other reflexes and thus partially reduces or blunts their effectiveness. However, the overall effect of an increase in renal artery pressure is still a net increase in sodium excretion (compare with Figure 7–7). GFR, glomerular filtration rate; P_{GC}, hydrostatic pressure in glomerular capillaries.

pressure and (2) the combined vascular resistances of the afferent and efferent arterioles, which determine how much of the arterial pressure is lost by the time the peritubular capillaries are reached. π_{PC} is set by (1) arterial oncotic pressure and (2) filtration fraction (GFR-RPF), which determine how much the oncotic pressure increases from its original arterial value during passage through the glomeruli.

Teleologically, it makes sense that P_{PC} and π_{PC} influence interstitial pressure and, hence, sodium reabsorption because these phenomena are simply a logical continuation

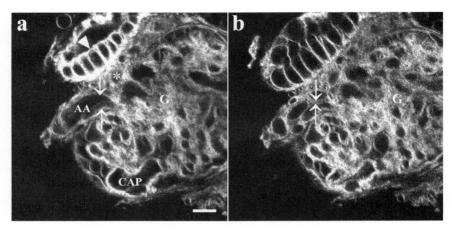

Figure 7–10. An example of tubuloglomerular feedback. Changes in juxtaglomerular apparatus morphology during increasing tubular NaCl concentration from 25 (osmolality = 210 mOsm/kg/H$_2$O) to 135 mmol (osmolality = 300 mOsm/kg/H$_2$O). Macula densa cell (arrowhead) swelling and parallel swelling/contraction of cells in the final part of the afferent arteriole causes an almost complete closure of the arteriolar lumen (arrows), collapse of capillary loops (CAP), and shrinkage of the entire glomerulus (G). *, mesangial cells. Bar = 10 μm. (From Peti-Peterdi J et al, Am J Physiol Renal Physiol 2002;283:F197. Used with permission.)

of the flow diagrams we have previously used for studying the homeostatic control of GFR. Events initiated by fluid loss end with 3 changes that lower GFR: increased constriction of the afferent and efferent arterioles (induced by the renal nerves and angiotensin II), decreased arterial hydraulic pressure, and increased arterial oncotic pressure. Figure 7–7 illustrates how these same 3 factors also decrease renal interstitial hydraulic pressure and, hence, increase sodium reabsorption. Thus, homeostatic responses that tend to lower GFR in response to a reduction in body sodium also usually increase sodium reabsorption, the "desired" homeostatic event, in response to bodily fluid depletion.

The same logic applies when the desired homeostatic responses are increased GFR and decreased sodium reabsorption so as to eliminate excess sodium from the body. Thus, when a high-salt diet or expansion of the ECF volume from some other physiological cause is the primary event, the following occurs: (1) decreased plasma oncotic pressure (resulting from dilution of plasma proteins), (2) increased arterial pressure, and (3) renal vasodilation secondary to decreased activity of the renal sympathetic nerves and decreased angiotensin II. (As already mentioned, however, this vasodilation may be very small or even nonexistent because the contribution of the renal nerves to renal vascular tone in a normal resting person is already so small that even complete elimination of it does not do much.) Simultaneously, then, the GFR increases a small amount and so does interstitial pressure, which reduces fluid reabsorption.

Glomerulotubular Balance

As stated earlier, in the regulation of sodium excretion, the control of tubular sodium *reabsorption* is more important than control of GFR. One reason for this is that a change in GFR automatically induces a proportional change in the reabsorption of sodium by the proximal tubules, so that the *fraction* reabsorbed (but not the total amount) remains relatively constant (Table 7–1). This phenomenon has the rather ungainly name of *glomerulotubular balance.* In response to a primary change in GFR, the percentage of the filtered sodium reabsorbed proximally remains approximately constant (about 65%). The fraction not reabsorbed also remains approximately constant (about 35%). Therefore, a change in GFR is still reflected as a change in the sodium and water presented to the loop of Henle. Glomerulotubular balance does not mean that proximal reabsorption is always exactly 65% of filtered sodium. It only says that when the fraction reabsorbed is changed, the change is caused by processes *other than* changes in GFR. Several mechanisms are manifested in the proximal tubule to stimulate sodium reabsorption (raise the percentage reabsorbed above 65%) or inhibit sodium reabsorption (lower the percentage below 65%).

The mechanisms responsible for matching changes in tubular reabsorption to changes in GFR are completely intrarenal (ie, glomerulotubular balance requires no external neural or hormonal input; indeed, the presence of such input usually obscures the existence of glomerulotubular balance, as described previously).

Glomerulotubular balance is actually a second line of defense preventing changes in renal hemodynamics per se from causing large changes in sodium excretion. The first line of defense is autoregulation of GFR, described in Chapter 2 and in the prior discussion of tubuloglomerular feedback. GFR autoregulation prevents GFR from changing too much in direct response to changes in blood pressure, and glomerulotubular balance blunts the sodium-excretion response to whatever GFR change does occur. Thus, tubuloglomerular feedback and glomerulotubular balance mediated by GFR autoregulation are processes that allow a large fraction of the responsibility for homeostatic control of sodium excretion to reside in those primary inputs that act to influence tubular reabsorption of sodium independently of GFR changes.

Table 7–1. Effect of "perfect" glomerulotubular balance on the mass of sodium leaving the proximal tubule

GFR (L/min)	P_{Na} (mmol/L)	Filtered (mmol/min)	Reabsorbed proximally (66.7% of filtered; mmol/min)	Leaving proximal (mmol/min)
0.124	145	18	12	6
0.165	145	24	16	8
0.062	145	9	6	3

The net result of fixed fractional reabsorption is to reduce the magnitude of difference in sodium leaving the proximal tubule.

CONTROL OF SODIUM BALANCE

As mentioned, pressure natriuresis and diuresis are effective at controlling ECF volume and, therefore, blood pressure. They are not particularly useful for *independently* controlling salt or water balance. Independent control of total body sodium balance requires additional specific hormonal mechanisms. Independent regulation of sodium reabsorption allows the mammalian kidney to compensate for the fact that, in terrestrial animals, sodium ingestion and water ingestion are both highly variable and often unrelated to each other.

Despite the necessity to alter sodium excretion independently of water excretion, maintaining sodium balance is still inextricably linked to blood pressure because, as mentioned, the primary variable that the kidney monitors is not total body sodium or plasma sodium but rather systemic blood pressure. However, unlike pressure diuresis and natriuresis, most of the processes for independent control of sodium balance occur in the *distal* nephron (not surprising because the distal nephron represents mammalian evolutionary adaptation to a terrestrial environment).

Aldosterone Regulation of Sodium Balance

In the face of a constant rate of ingestion of salt and water, correction of a sustained decrease in blood pressure requires a decrease in renal excretion of salt and water until the transient positive fluid balance returns blood volume to normal. A major control over the reabsorption of sodium in the distal nephron involves the hormone aldosterone. The primary effect of aldosterone is to increase sodium reabsorption in the connecting tubules and collecting ducts. The most important physiological factor controlling circulating levels of aldosterone is the circulating level of angiotensin II. Thus, a decrease in blood pressure produces a rapid short-term baroreceptor-mediated vascular response followed by the intermediate-term renal-mediated release of renin and production of angiotensin II, which reinforces the initial short-term vascular response. However, even if the blood pressure returns to near normal, the circulating angiotensin II will stimulate the adrenal cortex to produce aldosterone. This targets the distal nephron to increase sodium reabsorption and thus increase total body sodium and blood volume to produce a long-term correction to total body sodium content and mean blood pressure.

Aldosterone stimulates sodium reabsorption mainly by the cortical connecting tubule and cortical collecting duct, specifically by the principal cells, the same cells acted on by ADH. An action on this late portion of the nephron is what one would expect for fine-tuning the output of sodium, because more than 90% of the filtered sodium has already been reabsorbed by the time the filtrate reaches the collecting-duct system.

The total quantity of sodium reabsorption dependent on the influence of aldosterone is approximately 2% of the total filtered sodium. Thus, all other factors remaining constant, in the complete absence of aldosterone, a person would excrete 2% of the filtered sodium, whereas in the presence of maximal plasma concentrations of aldosterone, virtually no sodium would be excreted. Two percent of the filtered sodium may seem small but is actually large because of the huge volume of glomerular filtrate:

$$\begin{aligned} \text{Total filtered Na/day} &= \text{GFR} \times \text{PNa} \\ &= 180 \text{ L/day} \times 145 \text{ mmol/L} \\ &= 26{,}100 \text{ mmol/day} \end{aligned}$$

Thus, aldosterone controls the reabsorption of $0.02 \times 26{,}100$ mmol/day = 522 mmol/day. In terms of sodium chloride, the form in which most sodium is ingested, this amounts to approximately 30 g NaCl/day, an amount considerably more than the average person consumes. Therefore, by control of the plasma concentration of aldosterone between minimal and maximal, the excretion of sodium can be finely adjusted to the intake so that total-body sodium and ECF volume remain constant. (Interestingly, aldosterone also stimulates sodium transport by other epithelia in the body, namely, sweat and salivary ducts and the intestine. The net effect is the same as that exerted on the kidney: movement of sodium from lumen to blood. Thus, aldosterone is an all-purpose stimulator of sodium retention.) In the kidney, aldosterone acts like many other steroid hormones. As a molecule, it has enough lipid character to freely cross principal cell membranes, after which it combines with mineralocorticoid receptors in the cytoplasm. Aldosterone-bound receptors undergo a change in conformation that reveals a formerly hidden nuclear localization signal. After being transported to the nucleus, the receptor acts as a transcription factor that promotes gene expression and synthesis of messenger RNA (mRNA). The mRNA mediates translation of specific proteins. The effect of these proteins is to increase the activity or number of luminal membrane sodium channels and basolateral membrane Na-K-ATPase pumps to exactly what is needed to promote increased reabsorption of sodium (Figure 7–11).

Control of Aldosterone Secretion

Two major direct inputs to the adrenal gland stimulate aldosterone secretion and play a role in electrolyte balance (Figure 7–12): increased plasma potassium concentration and angiotensin II. In addition, the atrial natriuretic factors (discussed later) inhibit aldosterone secretion. The influence of plasma potassium concentration on aldosterone secretion is described in Chapter 8 in the context of the renal handling of potassium.

As described earlier, the plasma concentration of angiotensin II is determined mainly by the plasma concentration of renin. Accordingly, control of aldosterone secretion in sodium-regulating reflexes is determined by those factors that regulate renin secretion (ie, intrarenal baroreceptors, macula densa, and renal sympathetic nerves). Thus, when plasma volume is reduced, for example, by a low-sodium diet, hemorrhage, or diarrhea, renin secretion is stimulated, which leads, via angiotensin II, to an increased aldosterone secretion. This hormone then stimulates sodium reabsorption (Figure 7–13). In contrast, when a person ingests a high-sodium diet, renin secretion is reduced, which leads, via a reduced plasma angiotensin II, to decreased aldosterone secretion.

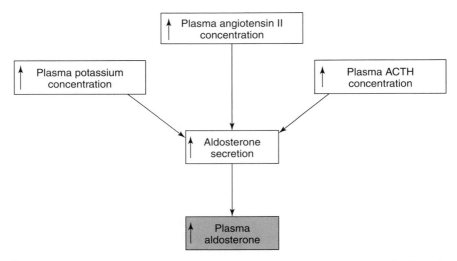

Figure 7–11. Mechanism of aldosterone action. Aldosterone enters principal cells and interacts with cytosolic aldosterone receptors. The aldosterone-bound receptors interact with nuclear DNA to promote gene expression. The aldosterone-induced gene products activate sodium channels and sodium pumps to increase sodium reabsorption. ACTH, adrenocorticotropic hormone.

Other Mechanisms for Controlling Sodium Balance

Although there are several other renal mechanisms for controlling sodium balance independent of water balance, under normal physiological circumstances none are as important as aldosterone. Only under certain pathophysiological conditions do these other mechanisms contribute significantly to regulation of sodium balance.

NATRIURETIC PEPTIDES

Several tissues in the body synthesize members of a hormone family called *natriuretic peptides,* so named because they promote excretion of sodium in the urine. Key among these are atrial natriuretic peptide (ANP) and brain natriuretic peptide (BNP; named as such because it was first discovered in the brain). The main source of both natriuretic peptides is the heart. The natriuretic peptides have both vascular and tubular actions. They relax the afferent arteriole, thereby promoting increased filtration, and act at several sites in the tubule. They inhibit release of renin, inhibit the actions of angiotensin II to promote reabsorption of sodium, and act in the medullary collecting duct to inhibit sodium absorption. The major stimulus for increased secretion of the natriuretic peptides is distention of the atria, which occurs during plasma volume expansion. This is probably the stimulus for the increased natriuretic peptides that occurs in persons on a high-salt diet (see Figure 7–6). Although most experts assume that these peptides play some physiological role in the regulation of sodium excretion in this and other situations in which plasma volume is expanded, it is not currently possible to quantitate precisely their contribution, although it is surely less than aldosterone.

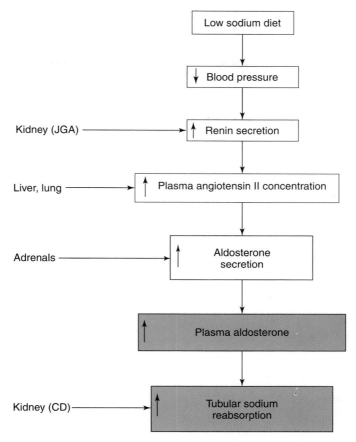

Figure 7–12. Regulation of plasma aldosterone. The major factors that determine circulating levels of aldosterone. Under normal conditions, the most important is angiotensin II and sometimes plasma potassium. Only angiotensin II produces a change in aldosterone that is directly related to maintaining sodium balance.

ANTIDIURETIC HORMONE

As described in Chapter 6, the major function of ADH is to increase the permeability of the cortical and medullary collecting ducts to water, thereby decreasing the excretion of water. In addition to this effect, ADH also increases sodium reabsorption by the cortical collecting duct, one of the same segments influenced by aldosterone. This effect is particularly evident when plasma aldosterone is elevated, and ADH's action seems to synergize with the action of this steroid hormone. This makes teleological sense because, as discussed later, the secretion of ADH, like that of aldosterone, is stimulated when plasma volume is reduced.

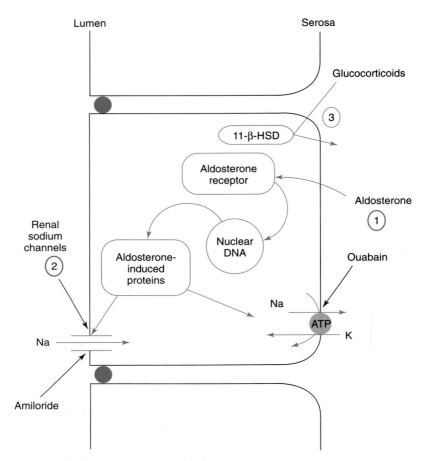

Figure 7–13. Factors that control aldosterone and sodium balance. JGA, juxtaglomerular apparatus; CD, collecting duct. 1. Abnormalities of the adrenals and certain tumors can lead to primary hyper- or hypoaldosteronism. 2. Loss of function mutations in sodium channels can lead to both pseudohypoaldosteronism; gain of function mutations produce pseudohyperaldosteronism (Liddle's syndrome). 3. Defects in 11β-hydroxysteroid dehydrogenase produces apparent mineralocorticoid excess because glucocorticoids can then interact with aldosterone receptors.

OTHER HORMONES

Many well-known hormones not normally associated with renal function can exert an influence on sodium reabsorption. Cortisol, estrogen, growth hormone, thyroid hormone, and insulin enhance sodium reabsorption, whereas glucagon, progesterone, and parathyroid hormone decrease it. When the level of any of these hormones is elevated (as, eg, of estrogen during pregnancy), it will exert a significant influence on sodium reabsorption and thus excretion. However, the secretion of these hormones, unlike the hormones described earlier, is not reflexively controlled specifically for the homeostatic regulation of sodium balance.

Summary of the Control of Sodium Excretion

The control of sodium excretion depends on the control of 2 variables of renal function: GFR and rate of sodium reabsorption (Tables 7–2 and 7–3). The latter is controlled by the renin-angiotensin-aldosterone hormonal system, renal sympathetic nerves, effects of arterial blood pressure on the kidneys (pressure natriuresis), and atrial natriuretic factors. The renal interstitial hydraulic pressure and several renal paracrine agents play important roles in regulating sodium reabsorption.

When considering mechanisms of sodium excretion, it is useful to consider 2 conceptually different categories of mechanisms: (1) proximal nephron mechanisms (control of GFR, pressure natriuresis, and, to a lesser extent, changes in Starling forces) that lead to coupled changes in sodium and water excretion and (2) distal nephron effects in which sodium can be reabsorbed independently of water. The proximal mechanisms are primarily involved in excreting excess ECF volume, whereas the distal mechanisms alter sodium excretion when ingestion of sodium is not balanced by ingestion of water. Both types of mechanisms can alter blood pressure because of the intimate relationship among total body sodium and water, blood volume, and blood pressure.

There is great flexibility in such a multifactor system. Thus, for example, although the renal sympathetic nerves influence GFR, renin secretion, renal interstitial hydraulic pressure, and the tubular cells themselves, a transplanted and, therefore,

Table 7–2. Effects of renal nerve stimulation

1	Stimulates renin secretion via a direct action on β_1-receptors of granular cells.
2	Stimulates sodium reabsorption via a direct action on tubular cells (multiple receptors); one site affected is the proximal tubule.
3	Stimulates afferent and efferent arteriolar constriction (α-adrenergic receptors).
	As a result:
a	GFR and RBF both decrease, the latter much more than the former.
b	The increased renal resistance decreases P_{PC}, and the increased filtration fraction increases π_{PC}. These changes cause renal interstitial hydraulic pressure to decrease, which stimulates sodium reabsorption, mainly in the proximal tubule.
c	The decreased GFR and the increased proximal sodium reabsorption (Effects 2 and 3b) result in decreased delivery of fluid to the macula densa, which causes increased renin secretion in addition to that of Effect 1 above.

The three categories of renal nerve effects are listed in the order in which they are elicited as the frequency of renal nerve impulses is increased to higher and higher values. Note that the direct effects on both renin secretion and sodium reabsorption occur at lower stimulation levels than those required to elicit renal vasoconstriction. GFR, glomerular filtration rate; RBF, renal blood flow; P_{PC}, peritubular-capillary hydraulic pressure; π_{PC}, peritubular capillary oncotic pressure.

Table 7–3. Changes in these factors influence sodium excretion in response to changes in plasma volume

Filtration of sodium
GFR
Plasma sodium concentration (of minor importance except in severe disorders)
Tubular reabsorption of sodium
Arterial blood pressure effects on proximal reabsorption (pressure natriuresis)
Aldosterone
Peritubular capillary factors, acting via RIHP
Renal nerves (direct tubular effects and indirect effects via angiotensin II and RIHP)
Angiotensin II (direct tubular effects and indirect effect via RIHP)
GFR (glomerotubular balance)
Atrial natriuretic factor
Antidiuretic hormone

GFR, glomerular filtration rate; RIHP, renal interstitial hydraulic pressure.

denervated kidney maintains sodium homeostasis quite well because of the other known *nonneural* factors involved. Overall, the one input whose absence causes the greatest difficulty in sodium regulation is aldosterone.

In normal persons, the mechanisms for regulating sodium excretion are so precise that sodium balance does not vary by more than a small percentage despite marked changes in dietary intake or losses caused by sweating, vomiting, diarrhea, hemorrhage, or burns.

CONTROL OF WATER EXCRETION

Water excretion, like sodium excretion, is the difference between the volume of water filtered (GFR) and the volume reabsorbed. Accordingly, the baroreceptor-initiated GFR-controlling reflexes described earlier tend to have the same effects on water excretion as on sodium excretion. As in the case of sodium, however, the major regulated determinant of water excretion is not the rate at which it is filtered but rather the rate at which it is reabsorbed. Also, as in the case of sodium excretion, water excretion conceptually consists of 2 major components: a proximal nephron component, in which water is absorbed along with sodium as an isotonic fluid, and a distal nephron component, in which water can be reabsorbed independent of sodium. The proximal nephron component is primarily a mechanism to regulate ECF volume in response to changes in blood pressure, and discussions of the factors that alter sodium reabsorption to produce pressure natriuresis also apply to water to produce pressure diuresis. As seen in Chapter 6, the *distal* nephron rate of water reabsorption (independent of sodium reabsorption) is determined mainly by ADH, which increases the water permeability of the collecting ducts, thereby increasing water reabsorption and, hence, decreasing water excretion. Accordingly, total-body water is regulated mainly by reflexes that alter the secretion of ADH.

ADH is a peptide produced by a discrete group of hypothalamic neurons whose cell bodies are located in the supraoptic and paraventricular nuclei and whose axons terminate in the posterior pituitary gland, from which ADH is released into the blood. The most important of the inputs to these neurons are from cardiovascular barore-ceptors and hypothalamic osmoreceptors.

Baroreceptor Control of ADH Secretion

A decreased extracellular volume (eg, resulting from diarrhea or hemorrhage) reflex-ively produces an increased aldosterone secretion. It also induces increased ADH secretion. The reflex is mediated by neural input to the ADH-secreting neurons from both cardiopulmonary and arterial baroreceptors.

Decreased cardiovascular pressures cause less firing by the baroreceptors. Via afferent neurons from the baroreceptors and ascending pathways to the hypothala-mus, this decreased baroreceptor firing causes stimulation of ADH secretion. Conversely, the baroreceptors are stimulated by increased cardiovascular pressures, and this causes inhibition of ADH secretion. The adaptive value of these baroreceptor reflexes is to help restore ECF volume and, hence, blood pressure (Figure 7–14).

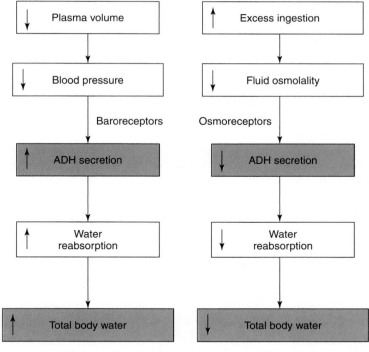

Figure 7–14. Regulation of water balance. The 2 major pathways for altering total body water. On the left, changes in antidiuretic hormone (ADH) release from the anterior pituitary are triggered by changes in blood volume. On the right, decreased osmolality causes swelling of osmoreceptor cells in the anterior hypothalamus, which inhibits their firing and inhibits adjacent superoptic nuclei cells that reduces ADH secretion from their axonal extensions in the posterior pituitary.

There is a second adaptive value to this reflex: Large decreases in plasma volume elicit, by way of the cardiovascular baroreceptors, such high concentrations of ADH—much higher than those needed to produce maximal antidiuresis—that the hormone is able to exert direct vasoconstrictor effects on arteriolar smooth muscle. The result is increased total peripheral resistance, which helps raise arterial blood pressure independently of the slower restoration of body fluid volumes. Renal arterioles and mesangial cells also participate in this constrictor response, and so a high plasma concentration of ADH, quite apart from its effect on tubular water permeability, may promote retention of both sodium and water by lowering GFR.

Osmoreceptor Control of ADH Secretion

We have seen how changes in ECF volume simultaneously elicit reflex changes in the excretion of both sodium and water. This is adaptive because the situations causing ECF volume alterations are often associated with loss or gain of both sodium and water in approximately proportional amounts. In contrast, we see now that changes in total-body water in which no change in total-body sodium occurs are compensated by alterations in water excretion but not in sodium excretion.

The major effect of gaining or losing water without corresponding changes in sodium is a change in the osmolality of the body fluids. This is a key point because, under conditions of predominantly water gain or loss, the receptors that initiate the reflexes controlling ADH secretion are osmoreceptors in the hypothalamus: receptors responsive to changes in osmolality. The hypothalamic cells that secrete ADH receive neural input from the osmoreceptors. Via these connections, an increase in osmolality stimulates them and increases their rate of ADH secretion. Conversely, decreased osmolality inhibits ADH secretion (see Figure 7–14). For example, when a person drinks 1 L of water, the excess water lowers the body fluid osmolality, which reflexively inhibits ADH secretion via the hypothalamic osmoreceptors. As a result, water permeability of the collecting ducts becomes very low, little or no water is reabsorbed from these segments, and a large volume of extremely dilute (hypoosmotic) urine is excreted. In this manner, the excess water is eliminated.

Conversely, when a pure-water deficit occurs (eg, because of water deprivation), the osmolality of the body fluids is increased, ADH secretion is reflexively stimulated, water permeability of the collecting ducts is increased, water reabsorption is maximal, and a very small volume of highly concentrated (hyperosmotic) urine is excreted. By this means, relatively less of the filtered water than solute is excreted, which is equivalent to adding pure water to the body, and the body fluid osmolality is restored toward normal.

We have described 2 different major afferent pathways controlling the ADH-secreting hypothalamic cells: one from baroreceptors and one from osmoreceptors. These hypothalamic cells are, therefore, true integrators, whose rate of activity is determined by the total synaptic input to them. Thus, a simultaneous increase in plasma volume and decrease in body fluid osmolality cause strong inhibition of ADH secretion. Conversely, a simultaneous decrease in plasma volume and increase in osmolality produce very marked stimulation of ADH secretion. However, what happens when baroreceptor and osmoreceptor inputs oppose each other (eg, if plasma volume and osmolality are both decreased)? In general, because of the high sensitivity of the osmoreceptors, the osmoreceptor influence predominates over that of the baroreceptor when changes in osmolality and plasma volume are small to moderate. However, a very large change in plasma volume will take precedence over decreased body fluid osmolality in influencing ADH secretion; under such conditions, water is retained in excess of solute, and the body fluids become hypo-osmotic (for the same reason, plasma sodium concentration decreases). In essence, it is more important for the body to preserve vascular volume and thus ensure an adequate cardiac output than it is to preserve normal osmolality.

The ADH-secreting cells also receive synaptic input from many other brain areas. Thus, ADH secretion and, hence, urine flow can be altered by pain, fear, and a variety of other factors, including drugs such as alcohol, which inhibits ADH release. However, this complexity should not obscure the generalization that ADH secretion is determined over the long term primarily by the states of body fluid osmolality and plasma volume.

Several diseases (eg, diabetes insipidus, which is different from diabetes mellitus, also known as sugar diabetes) illustrate what happens when the ADH system is disrupted. Diabetes insipidus is characterized by a constant water diuresis, as much as 25 L/day. In most cases, people with diabetes insipidus have lost the ability to produce ADH because of damage to the hypothalamus or have lost the ability to respond to ADH because of defects in principal cell ADH receptors. Thus, collecting-duct permeability to water is low and unchanging regardless of extracellular osmolality or volume. In contrast, other diseases (eg, head trauma or brain tumors) are associated with inappropriately large secretion of ADH. As is predictable, patients with these diseases manifest decreased plasma osmolality (and sodium concentration) because of the excessive reabsorption of pure water.

Figure 7–15 summarizes the major factors known to control renal sodium and water excretion in response to severe sweating. Sweat is a hypo-osmotic solution containing mainly water, sodium, and chloride. Therefore, sweating causes both a decrease in ECF volume and an increase in body fluid osmolality. The renal retention of water and sodium helps to compensate for the water and salt lost in the sweat.

Thirst and Salt Appetite

Large deficits of salt and water can be only partly compensated by renal conservation of these substances, and ingestion is the ultimate compensatory mechanism. The centers that mediate thirst are located in the hypothalamus (very close to those areas that produce ADH). The subjective feeling of thirst, which drives one to obtain and ingest water, is stimulated both by reduced plasma volume and by increased body fluid osmolality. The adaptive significance of both are self-evident. Note that these are precisely the same changes that stimulate ADH production, and the receptors—osmoreceptors and the nerve cells that respond to the cardiovascular baroreceptors—that initiate the ADH-controlling reflexes are near those that initiate thirst. The thirst response, however, is significantly less sensitive than the ADH response.

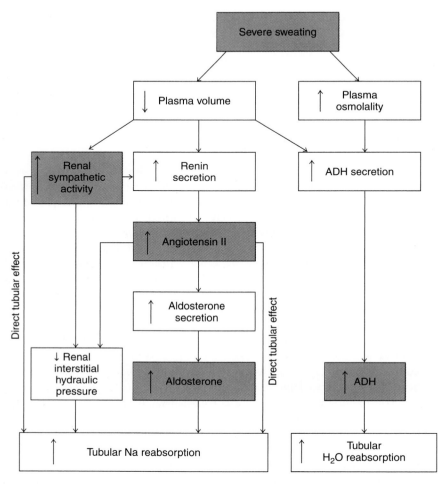

Figure 7–15. Summary of major factors that increase tubular sodium and water reabsorption in severe sweating. (Antidiuretic hormone [ADH] also enhances sodium reabsorption, but this is a relatively minor effect and is not shown.) These changes, coupled with the decrease in GFR that also occurs, homeostatically reduce urinary sodium and water loss. (To visualize the response to a high-sodium diet or the infusion of saline, simply replace "severe sweating" with these events, reverse all the arrows in the boxes, and add an increase in atrial natriuretic peptide, the result of atrial distention.)

There are also other pathways controlling thirst. For example, dryness of the mouth and throat causes profound thirst, which is relieved by merely moistening them. Also, when animals such as the camel (and humans, to a lesser extent) become markedly dehydrated, they will rapidly drink just enough water to replace their previous losses and then stop. What is amazing is that when they stop, the water has not yet had time to be absorbed from the gastrointestinal tract into the blood. Some kind of metering of the water intake by the gastrointestinal tract has occurred, but its nature remains a mystery.

Angiotensin II is yet another factor that stimulates thirst: by its direct effect on the brain. This hormone constitutes one of the pathways by which thirst is stimulated when ECF volume is decreased.

Salt appetite, which is the analogue of thirst, is also an extremely important component of sodium homeostasis in most mammals. It is clear that salt appetite in these species is innate and consists of 2 components: (1) hedonistic appetite and (2) regulatory appetite. In other words, (1) animals like salt and eat it whenever they can regardless of whether they are salt deficient, and (2) their drive to obtain salt is markedly increased in the presence of deficiency.

The significance of these animal studies for humans, however, is unclear. Salt craving does seem to occur in humans who are severely salt depleted, but the contribution of such regulatory salt appetite to everyday sodium homeostasis in normal persons is probably slight. On the other hand, humans do seem to have a strong hedonistic appetite for salt, as manifested by almost universally large intakes of sodium whenever it is cheap and readily available. Thus, the average American intake of salt is 10–15 g/day even though humans can survive quite normally on less than 0.5 g/day. As pointed out previously, a large salt intake may be a contributor to the pathogenesis of hypertension in susceptible individuals.

Congestive Heart Failure and Hypertension: Cardiovascular Pathologies That Involve Altered Sodium Excretion

Congestive heart failure and hypertension involve perturbed renal handling of sodium. In congestive heart failure and in most cases of hypertension, the perturbed renal function seems to lie in inappropriate *signaling* to the kidneys rather than pathology of renal transport mechanisms per se.

Congestive heart failure is characterized by weak cardiac muscle that cannot increase cardiac output to meet the demands of exercise and, more importantly, can only provide an adequate resting cardiac output in the presence of excessive neurohumoral drive (something like a car operating on 2 cylinders that can only keep up speed when the accelerator is pushed to the floor). The neurohumoral drive is characterized by high levels of renin, angiotensin II, aldosterone, catecholamines, and other mediators. Fluid volume is increased, leading to edema in the lungs, peripheral tissues, or both, which is why this is called *congestive* heart failure. Because of the high fluid volume, atrial pressures sensed by the cardiopulmonary baroreceptors are high. The high atrial pressures should lead to decreased ADH secretion and decreased sympathetic drive to the kidneys.[5] Instead, these signals are *increased,* and the kidneys operate at a new setpoint in which normal sodium excretion only occurs

---

[5] In contrast to atrial pressures that are high, *arterial* pressure is usually within the normal range, and heart failure cannot be diagnosed based on arterial blood pressure. It may be that arterial pressure is actually a little below the setpoint of the brainstem vasomotor center, leading to the sympathetic drive associated with heart failure. However, there is no way to measure the setpoint and compare it with the pressures that actually exist in the arterial tree.

at the expense of an excessive body fluid volume. If fluid volume is somehow restored to normal levels, renal excretion of sodium drops to very low levels. Another characteristic of congestive heart failure is high levels of natriuretic peptides. This is an appropriate response to the high atrial pressures and partially counteracts the sodium-retaining signals to the kidneys but does not restore sodium output to a level that would occur in a healthy person who transiently developed the high fluid volume that exists chronically in the heart failure patient. The high fluid volumes of congestive heart failure are deleterious to pulmonary function and over time often lead to structural changes in the heart (dilation) that only exacerbate the defective pumping. Therapy for congestive heart failure includes the use of diuretics to reduce the high fluid volume and drugs that inhibit the generation of angiotensin II (ACE inhibitors) or block the actions of angiotensin II (angiotensin receptor antagonists).

Hypertension is also a disease of abnormal sodium balance. Hypertension must always be associated with a blood volume and total body sodium content that is too high for the volume of the vascular tree. In some cases, the reason for the excess blood volume is clear. For example, renal glomerular disease often leads to inappropriate release of renin with subsequent increases in angiotensin II, aldosterone, collecting-tubule sodium reabsorption, and finally an increase in blood pressure; a tumor of the adrenal cortex can lead to excess production of aldosterone and increases in blood pressure; or a specific gain of function mutation in the sodium reabsorptive mechanism in the collecting duct also leads to excess sodium reabsorption and profound hypertension. These 3 examples illustrate 3 types of defects in the complicated control mechanism for maintaining total body sodium and mean blood pressure. The first, excess renin production, is a problem with the sensing mechanism for the renal component of the blood pressure control system. The second, excess production of aldosterone, is a defect in the signaling mechanism that lies between the sensor (pressure sensors in the large vessels and the kidney) and the effector (distal nephron sodium reabsorption). The third example is a defect in the effector system (distal nephron sodium reabsorption). In these cases, the defect is more or less obvious, and correcting the underlying pathology usually corrects the hypertension (ie, ACE inhibitors reduce the effect of excess renin, spironolactone will inhibit aldosterone receptors, and administration of amiloride will reduce sodium reabsorption by epithelial sodium channels). Table 7–4 provides a list of identifiable genetic defects in the regulation of sodium balance that lead to either increases or decreases in blood pressure. Despite the relatively extensive list of known defects, in many cases of hypertension, the cause is unclear. Renin levels, angiotensin levels, and aldosterone levels are normal or even reduced, and yet blood pressure is elevated as if the setpoint of the control loop from sensing blood pressure to sodium reabsorption is inexplicably high. The relatively normal levels of circulating renin, angiotensin II, and aldosterone imply that the defect in the regulation of sodium reabsorption lies subsequent to aldosterone interaction with the cells of the collecting tubule. One holy grail of hypertension research has been to define the components responsible for controlling sodium reabsorption that are induced by aldosterone in an effort to intervene in the process that leads to increased total body sodium and increased blood pressure.

Table 7–4. Genetic bases for changes in blood pressure

Syndrome	Defect	Characteristics
Hypertension		
Apparent mineralocorticoid excess (AME)	Loss of function mutation of 11β-hydroxysteroid dehydrogenase	Aldosterone receptors in renal principal cells not only are activated by aldosterone, but can be activated by normal levels of circulating glucocorticoids promoting constitutive sodium reabsorption with profound early-onset hypertension and growth arrest. Responsive to mineralocorticoid (aldosterone) receptor antagonists (eg, spironolactone, eplerenone).
Liddle's syndrome	Gain of function mutation in the β or γ subunit of ENaC	Constitutive sodium reabsorption regardless of circulating aldosterone levels with profound early-onset hypertension. Responsive to amiloride (Midamor).
T594M β-ENaC	Single amino acid mutation in β subunit of ENaC with moderate gain of function	Increased collecting-duct sodium reabsorption with mild to moderate hypertension. Most prevalent in individuals of African descent. Responsive to amiloride (Midamor).
Glucocorticoid-remediable aldosteronism	Elevated aldosterone resulting from an abnormal activation of aldosterone synthase by ACTH	Early-onset hypertension that can be controlled by administration of glucocorticoids (to reduce ACTH production).
Aldosterone synthase polymorphisms	Gain of function leading to increased circulating aldosterone	Increased sodium reabsorption with mild hypertension. Most prevalent in men. More prevalent in individuals of Japanese descent. Responsive to mineralocorticoid (aldosterone) receptor antagonists (eg, spironolactone, eplerenone).

(Continued)

Table 7–4. Genetic bases for changes in blood pressure (*Continued*)

Syndrome	Defect	Characteristics
11β-hydroxylase deficiency	Loss of function mutation leading to abnormal accumulation of 11-deoxycorticosterone, which activates aldosterone receptors	Activation of aldosterone receptors leads to sodium retention and early-onset hypertension. Associated accumulation of androgens leads to masculinization of females in utero and both sexes postnatally. May be responsive to the aldosterone receptor antagonist eplerenone, but spironolactone would exacerbate androgenic effects.
Pseudohypoaldosteronism type II (Gordon's syndrome)	Loss of function mutation in WNK kinases	Loss of WNK function leads to activation of distal nephron thiazide-sensitive sodium chloride cotransporter causing sodium retention, hypertension, and hyperkalemia. Responsive to thiazides.
α-adducin polymorphism	Structural protein that activates Na-K-ATPase	Increased Na pump activity modestly increases sodium reabsorption to produce mild hypertension.
Hypertension exacerbated in pregnancy	Mutation in mineralocorticoid receptor that makes receptor more sensitive to aldosterone	Early-onset hypertension greatly exaggerated by pregnancy because progesterone also binds to the mutant receptor and promotes additional sodium reabsorption. The aldosterone receptor antagonist spironolactone acts as an agonist for the mutant receptor; effect of eplerenone has not been examined.
SGK	Two activating mutations	SGK inhibits ENaC degradation so activation causes accumulation of ENaC and an increase in renal sodium reabsorption with consequent hypertension. Possibly responsive to amiloride (Midamor).

Table 7–4. Genetic bases for changes in blood pressure (*Continued*)

Syndrome	Defect	Characteristics
Various SNPs in the genes for renin, ACE, and angiotensin II receptor	Presumably slightly altered function of the genes controlling angiotensin production and sensitivity	Statistically significant increases in blood pressure. Some SNPs are more prevalent in African Americans, others more prevalent in European Americans, and a few prevalent in both populations. Responsive to ACE inhibitors (eg, captopril, benazepril [Lotensin]) and angiotensin II receptor inhibitors (eg, losartan), and volume reduction with thiazide diuretics.
Hypotension		
Pseudohypoaldosteronism type I (dominant)	Loss of function mutation of the mineralocorticoid receptor	Salt wasting, hypotension, severe neonatal symptoms.
Pseudohypoaldosteronism type I (recessive)	Partial loss of function mutation of the α subunit of ENaC	Salt wasting, hypotension, hyperkalemia, excess fluid secretion from airways, loss of salt taste, serious symptoms at all ages.
Aldosterone synthase	Loss of function leading to decreased circulating aldosterone	Decreased sodium reabsorption with severe hypotension and occasionally shock because of reduced intravascular volume.
Steroid 21-hydroxylase	Loss of function leading to decreased synthesis of aldosterone	Decreased sodium reabsorption with severe hypotension and other endocrine abnormalities.
Gitelman's syndrome	Loss of function of distal nephron thiazide-sensitive NaCl transporter	Salt wasting and mild hypotension in homozygotes.

ACTH, advenocorticotropic hormone; WNK, *with, no* kinase (lysine); ATPase, adenosine triphosphatase; SGK, serum and glucocorticoid-regulated kinase; SNP, single nucleotide polymorphism; ACE, angiotensin-converting enzyme.

KEY CONCEPTS

Multiple overlapping mechanisms regulate sodium and water excretion; most are related to blood pressure.

The medullary vasomotor center regulates blood pressure on a moment-to moment basis via the baroreceptor reflex and also regulates renal excretion of sodium and water.

The kidneys have their own means of regulating sodium excretion independent of vasomotor control; key among these are pressure natriuresis and the renin-angiotensin system.

The kidneys are the ultimate determinant of blood pressure in the long term via their control of ECF volume.

All the physiological controls in the proximal nephron affect the excretion of sodium and water together, whereas the actions of aldosterone and ADH in the distal nephron regulate sodium and water excretion independently.

Long-term regulation of sodium excretion and, therefore, blood pressure centers on the actions of aldosterone.

ADH secretion is regulated both by blood pressure, via the baroreceptor-vasomotor center system, and plasma osmolality via hypothalamic osmoreceptors.

STUDY QUESTIONS

7–1. *In a canine experiment, a dog's filtered load of sodium in an isolated pump-perfused kidney is found to be 15 mmol/min. (1) How much sodium do you predict remains in the tubule at the end of the proximal tubule? (2) If its GFR is suddenly increased by 33%, how much sodium now is left at the end of the proximal tubule?*

7–2. *Normally aldosterone stimulates the reabsorption of approximately 33 g of sodium chloride/day. If a patient loses 100% of adrenal function, will 33 g of sodium chloride be excreted per day indefinitely?*

7–3. *A patient has suffered a severe hemorrhage and the plasma protein concentration is normal. (Not enough time has elapsed for interstitial fluid to move into the plasma.) Does this mean that the peritubular-capillary oncotic pressure is also normal?*

7–4. *If the right renal artery becomes abnormally constricted, what will happen to renin secretion by the right kidney and the left kidney?*

7–5. *A patient is suffering from primary hyperaldosteronism (ie, increased secretion of aldosterone caused by an aldosterone-producing adrenal tumor). Is plasma renin concentration higher or lower than normal?*

7–6. An agent that increases sodium and water excretion is called a diuretic (even though natriuretic is probably a better term). Block of sodium reabsorption in the proximal tubule, loop of Henle, distal tubule, or collecting duct will exert a diuretic effect. True or false?

7–7. A person is given a drug that dilates both the afferent and efferent arterioles. Assuming no other action of the drug, what will happen to the percentage of filtered sodium that this person's proximal tubule reabsorbs?

7–8. A new drug is found to have dual actions: It blocks sodium entry pathways in the proximal tubule epithelium, and it binds to ADH receptors in the collecting ducts and mimics the actions of ADH. Will the final urine contain excess or low amounts of sodium and excess or low amounts of water, and will it be hyperosmotic, iso-osmotic, or hypo-osmotic?

7–9. Another new drug also has dual actions, this time blocking sodium entry pathways in the thick ascending limb and exerting ADH-like actions as in Question 7–8. Now will the final urine contain excess or low amounts of sodium and excess or low amounts of water, and will it be hyperosmotic, iso-osmotic, or hypo-osmotic?

SUGGESTED READING

Cowley AW Jr, Liard JF, Guyton AC. Role of baroreceptor reflex in daily control of arterial blood pressure and other variables in dogs. *Circ Res* 1973;32:564.

Renal Regulation of Potassium Balance

8

OBJECTIVES

The student understands the internal exchanges of potassium:

▶ States the normal balance and distribution of potassium within different body compartments, including cells and extracellular fluid.

▶ Describes how potassium moves between cells and the extracellular fluid, and how, on a short-term basis, the movement protects the extracellular fluid from large changes in potassium concentration.

▶ Describes how plasma levels of potassium do not always reflect the status of total-body potassium.

The student understands the renal regulation of potassium excretion:

▶ States generalizations about renal potassium handling for persons on high- or low-potassium diets.

▶ States the relative amounts of potassium reabsorbed by the proximal tubule and thick ascending limb of Henle's loop regardless of the state of potassium intake.

▶ Describes how the cortical collecting duct can manifest net secretion or reabsorption; describes the role of principal cells and intercalated cells in these processes.

▶ Lists the 3 inputs that control the rate of potassium secretion by the cortical collecting duct.

▶ Describes the mechanism by which changes in potassium balance influence aldosterone secretion.

▶ States the effects of most diuretic drugs and osmotic diuretics on potassium excretion.

▶ Describes the association between perturbations in acid-base status and the plasma potassium level.

Potassium, like all other important ions, is distributed between the intracellular fluid and extracellular fluid (ECF) of the body.

The vast majority is intracellular, and only about 2% of the total potassium is extracellular. This small fraction, however, is absolutely crucial for body function, and the concentration of potassium in the ECF is a closely regulated quantity. Major elevations and depressions (called *hyperkalemia* and *hypokalemia*) away from the normal value of 4 mEq/L are cause for medical intervention. The importance of maintaining this concentration relatively constant stems primarily from the role of potassium in the excitability of nerve and muscle. The resting membrane potentials of these tissues are strongly influenced by the ratio of intracellular to extracellular potassium concentration. Raising the extracellular potassium concentration depolarizes the resting membrane potential, thus perturbing cell excitability. Conversely, lowering the extracellular potassium concentration usually hyperpolarizes cell membranes.[1]

REGULATION OF POTASSIUM BETWEEN THE INTRACELLULAR AND EXTRACELLULAR COMPARTMENTS

Given that the vast majority of body potassium is within cells, the extracellular potassium concentration is crucially dependent on (1) the total amount of potassium in the body and (2) the *distribution* of this potassium between the extracellular and intracellular fluid compartments. Total-body potassium is determined by the balance between potassium intake and excretion. Normal individuals remain in potassium balance, as they do in sodium balance, by excreting an amount of urinary potassium equal to the amount of potassium ingested minus the small amounts eliminated in the feces and sweat. Normally, potassium losses via sweat and the gastrointestinal tract are small, but very large quantities can be lost from the tract during vomiting or diarrhea. Again, the control of renal function is the major mechanism by which total-body potassium is maintained in balance.

The fact that most body potassium is intracellular follows strictly from the size and properties of the intracellular and extracellular compartments. About two thirds of the body fluids are intracellular (the collective cytosolic volume of all the cells in the body); typical cytosolic potassium concentrations are about 140–150 mEq/L. One third of the body fluids are extracellular, with a potassium concentration of about 4 mEq/L. In a clinical setting, only the extracellular concentration can be measured (the intracellular potassium is, in a sense, hidden behind the wall of the cell membrane). Furthermore, the extracellular value does not necessarily reflect total-body potassium. A patient may, for example, be hyperkalemic (high plasma potassium concentration) and yet at the same time be depleted of total-body potassium.

The high level of potassium within cells is maintained by the collective operation of the sodium-potassium-adenosine triphosphatase (Na-K-ATPase) plasma membrane pumps, which actively transport potassium into cells. Because the amount of potassium in the extracellular compartment is so small, even very slight shifts of potassium into or out of cells can produce large changes in extracellular potassium concentration. Such shifts, particularly in muscle, which makes up the largest store of potassium in the body, are to some extent under physiological control. Therefore, when extracellular potassium concentration changes because of either changes in total-body

---

[1] Whether a given change in potassium concentration makes an excitable cell more or less excitable is not always obvious. Depolarization resulting from elevated extracellular potassium *may* make a cell more excitable, but very strong depolarization actually decreases excitability (because of inactivation of voltage-gated sodium channels), a situation called a *depolarizing block*. In cases of very high extracellular potassium, a depolarizing block in the heart prevents propagation of the electrical signal that causes synchronized contraction.

potassium (ie, imbalances between intake and excretion) or internal shifts between the intracellular and extracellular compartments secondary to other events (eg, cell damage), potassium moves into or out of muscle cells, effectively buffering the extracellular concentration. On a moment-to-moment basis, this is what protects the ECF from large swings in potassium concentration. Major factors involved in these homeostatic processes include epinephrine and insulin, both of which cause increased potassium uptake by muscle (and certain other cells) through stimulation of plasma-membrane Na-K-ATPase.

The effect of epinephrine on cellular potassium uptake is probably of greatest physiological importance during exercise and trauma. In exercise, potassium moves out of muscle cells that are rapidly firing action potentials, and damaged cells leak potassium. In both cases, this raises extracellular potassium concentration.[2] However, at the same time, exercise or trauma increases adrenal secretion of epinephrine, and this hormone's stimulation of potassium uptake by other cells partially offsets the outflow from the exercising or damaged cells.

The rise in plasma insulin concentration after a meal is an important factor in moving ingested and absorbed potassium into cells rather than allowing it to accumulate in the ECF. This new potassium then slowly comes out of cells between meals to be excreted. Moreover, a large increase in plasma potassium concentration facilitates insulin secretion at any time, and the additional insulin induces greater potassium uptake by the cells, a negative feedback system for opposing acute elevations in plasma potassium concentration. In the natural order of things, insulin also stimulates glucose uptake and metabolism by cells: a necessary source of energy to drive the insulin-activated Na-K-ATPase responsible for moving potassium into cells.

Still another influence on the distribution of potassium between the intracellular fluid and ECF is the ECF hydrogen ion concentration: An increase in ECF hydrogen ion concentration (acidosis; see Chapter 9) is often associated with net potassium movement out of cells, whereas a decrease in ECF hydrogen ion concentration (alkalosis) causes net potassium movement into them. It is as though potassium and hydrogen ions were exchanging across plasma membranes (ie, hydrogen ions moving into the cell during acidosis and out during alkalosis and potassium doing just the opposite), but the precise mechanism underlying these "exchanges" has not yet been clarified. However, like the effect of insulin, it probably involves an inhibition (acidosis) or activation (alkalosis) of the Na-K-ATPase.

RENAL POTASSIUM HANDLING

Overview

The renal handling of potassium is, not surprisingly, rather complicated. Potassium is freely filtered, and the majority is immediately reabsorbed in the proximal tubule.

---

[2] During very intense intermittent exercise (eg, wind sprints), extracellular potassium can easily double as a result of release from exercising muscle. As soon as exercise stops, the muscle takes it back up rapidly, within 1 minute or so. Without the influence of catecholamine hormones on sensitive tissues such as the heart, the suddenly high levels of potassium reached during intense exercise would be quite dangerous.

Most of the rest is reabsorbed in the loop of Henle, so that under virtually all conditions only about 10% of the filtered load is presented to the distal nephron (ie, regions beyond the thick ascending limb). In the collecting ducts, reabsorption is continuous.

Under conditions of a low-potassium diet, this reabsorption is the dominant process, so that only a small fraction (less than 5% of the filtered load) is excreted. However, the collecting ducts also have the capacity to secrete potassium. When the diet is high in potassium, the secretory process is stimulated, and the secretory rate becomes much higher than the ongoing reabsorptive rate. Because secretion exceeds reabsorption, potassium is excreted; in some conditions, the excreted amount is actually greater than the filtered load. The key regulated variable in all of this is the rate of secretion by the collecting ducts. When it is high, large amounts of potassium are excreted. When low, the ongoing reabsorption reclaims most of the potassium, and little is excreted.

The tubular handling of potassium is summarized in Table 8–1. As mentioned, regardless of an individual's bodily potassium status, the proximal tubule reabsorbs approximately 60–80% of filtered potassium and the thick ascending limb of Henle's loop about 10–20%, leaving 10% or so to be passed on to the distal nephron. The mechanisms for potassium reabsorption in these 2 segments are understandable based on our prior discussions of ion transport. First, reabsorption in the proximal tubule is mainly by paracellular diffusion, the concentration gradient for which is created, as for urea and chloride, by water reabsorption (ie, as water is reabsorbed, this concentrates any solutes remaining in the lumen). Second, reabsorption in the thick ascending limb is mainly driven by the luminal membrane Na-K-2Cl

Table 8–1. Summary of tubular potassium transport

Transport	Normal- or high-potassium diet	Low-potassium diet or potassium depletion
Proximal tubule	Reabsorption (60–80%)	Reabsorption (55%)
Thick ascending limb	Reabsorption (5–25%)	Reabsorption (30%)
Distal convoluted tubule	Secretion	Reabsorption
Principal cells, cortical collecting duct	Substantial secretion (> 15%)	Little secretion
H-K-ATPase-containing intercalated cells, cortical collecting duct	Reabsorption (10%)	Reabsorption (10%)
H-K-ATPase-containing cells, medullary collecting duct	Reabsorption (5%)	Reabsorption (5%)

Percentages are in reference to the filtered load of potassium. H, hydrogen; K, potassium, ATPase, adenosine triphosphatase.

multiporter[3] (see Figure 6–3) and partially by paracellular diffusion. Because the multiporter requires the operation of the basolateral Na-K-ATPase to keep cytosolic sodium low (and because water reabsorption in the proximal tubule also depends on the Na-K-ATPase), potassium reabsorption is ultimately dependent on sodium reabsorption.[4]

What about the rest of the tubule (Table 8–1)? For an individual who is on a low-potassium diet or is potassium depleted for some other reason, the distal segments reabsorb potassium. The end result is that only a very small amount of potassium is excreted.

In contrast, for an individual on a normal or high-potassium diet, the distal convoluted tubule and the cortical collecting duct both manifest net potassium secretion, and the amount of potassium in the tubule increases markedly. The greater an individual's potassium intake or positive bodily potassium balance, the greater is the amount of potassium secreted by these segments. The final tubular segment, the medullary collecting duct, still reabsorbs potassium. However, when large amounts of potassium are being secreted upstream, the reabsorption only succeeds in recovering a small amount of that entering the medullary lumen. The overall result, therefore, of the various tubular contributions in individuals on a normal- or high-potassium diet is that the great majority of the excreted potassium is potassium that was secreted by the distal convoluted tubule and cortical collecting duct.

Because the contribution (either reabsorptive or secretory) of the cortical collecting duct is much greater than that of the distal convoluted tubule, we refer only to it in the remainder of this chapter. How is it that the cortical collecting duct can manifest either net reabsorption or net secretion? Recall once again that the collecting-duct system contains a mixture of cell types: principal cells and intercalated cells.

It is the principal cells—the same cells we described earlier as the aldosterone-regulated reabsorbers of sodium and the antidiuretic hormone-regulated reabsorbers of water—that secrete potassium. In contrast, the intercalated cells—specifically Type A—reabsorb potassium. (This reabsorptive process also mediates the simultaneous tubular secretion of hydrogen ions and is described in Chapter 9). Under conditions of normal or high potassium intake, principal cell potassium secretion is much greater than potassium reabsorption by Type A intercalated cells, and so the cortical collecting duct shows net secretion. During potassium depletion, however, the principal cells reduce their secretion, and so, on balance, there is net reabsorption.

Thus, the renal handling of potassium may be summarized by the following important generalization (see Table 8–1): Differences in potassium excretion over the

---

[3] As discussed in Chapter 6, much of the potassium entering the cytosol via the multiporter leaks via potassium channels back into the lumen and is recycled. This provides an available supply of potassium to accompany the sodium moving on the multiporter.

[4] Although the loops of Henle as a whole exhibit net reabsorption, long loops of Henle (from juxtamedullary nephrons) secrete potassium in the thin descending limb; this potassium comes from the medullary interstitium. In turn, interstitial potassium comes from potassium reabsorption in the medullary collecting ducts. Thus, there is some potassium recycling analogous to the urea recycling described earlier.

usual physiological range are due primarily to differences in the amount of potassium *secreted* by the cortical collecting duct. It is this variable that is controlled to regulate urinary potassium excretion. There is little, if any, homeostatic control over potassium reabsorption in any tubular segment.

This secretory process is so dominant in determining changes in potassium excretion that, in describing the control of potassium excretion, we tend to ignore any contribution of changes in either filtered potassium or tubular transport before the collecting-duct system. It must be pointed out, however, that under certain conditions potassium reabsorption in the proximal tubule or Henle's loop may be decreased (eg, in Bartter's syndrome, which is caused by a loss of function mutation in the Na-K-2Cl symporter in the thick ascending limb). Thus, a large quantity of the potassium excreted may represent filtered potassium that has not been reabsorbed. The most frequent problem of this sort in a medical setting is due to diuretics that inhibit sodium reabsorption by the proximal tubule or thick ascending limb of Henle's loop that also inhibit potassium reabsorption at these sites. The reasons should be clear from the sodium dependence of potassium reabsorption in these segments. Osmotic diuretics, predictably, interfere with potassium reabsorption in these segments, which is one reason for the marked urinary loss of potassium among patients with uncontrolled diabetes mellitus who have large amounts of filtered and unreabsorbed glucose.

Mechanism of Potassium Secretion in the Cortical Collecting Duct

As discussed, differences in potassium excretion over the usual physiological range are due primarily to differences in the amount of potassium *secreted* by the principal cells of the cortical collecting duct. Figure 8–1 summarizes the pathway for potassium secretion in these cells. This secretion involves active transport of potassium into the cell across the basolateral membrane and passive exit across the luminal membrane. The critical event is the active transport of potassium from interstitial fluid across the basolateral membrane into the cell. This active transport step, which is mediated via Na-K-ATPase pumps, continuously puts potassium into these cells. This potassium must either leak back to the interstitium or be secreted into the lumen. In this case, it moves into the lumen through the numerous luminal potassium channels in this tubular segment. The principal cells also express K-Cl symporters in their luminal membranes, and some potassium moves into the lumen via this pathway.

Homeostatic Control of Potassium Secretion by the Cortical Collecting Duct

How is the potassium secretion by principal cells of the cortical collecting duct regulated to achieve homeostasis of body potassium? Current understanding of potassium homeostasis suggests that there are 3 key factors: (1) the concentration of potassium in the blood perfusing the kidney, (2) plasma levels of aldosterone, and (3) the delivery of sodium to the distal nephron. When a large amount of potassium is ingested, most is rapidly taken up by cells all over the body (particularly muscle). This is probably due to increased activity of the Na-K-ATPase (after all, one substrate for the Na-K-ATPase is potassium, so that an increase in blood levels of potassium should

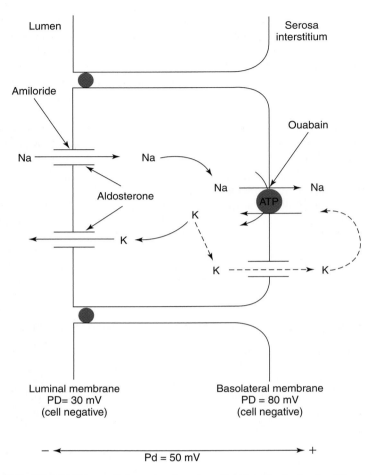

Figure 8–1. Model of transcellular potassium secretion by principal cells of the cortical collecting duct. (Although not indicated, there is an effect on Na-K-ATPase if aldosterone levels remain high for a sufficient period of time [days to weeks].) Potassium is actively moved into the cell by the basolateral membrane Na-K-ATPase pumps and then diffuses across the luminal membranes through potassium channels (ROMK). Note that there is also some potassium diffusion back across basolateral membrane channels from the cell into the interstitial fluid; this is "wasted" potassium so far as potassium secretion is concerned. The amount is small, however, compared with movement through the luminal membrane potassium channels because of the differences in electrical potentials across the 2 membranes and the much smaller number of potassium channels in the basolateral membrane. Both the reabsorption of sodium and secretion of potassium by these cells is regulated by aldosterone. ATP, adenosine triphosphate; PD, potassium diffusion.

promote increased activity; ie, increased potassium uptake by cells). The principal cells of the cortical collecting duct are no exception. They contain an isoform of the Na-K-ATPase that is especially sensitive to increases in the concentration of potassium in the peritubular capillaries and increase their uptake of potassium as the basolateral Na-K-ATPase is activated. The resulting increase in intracellular potassium concentration enhances the concentration gradient for potassium movement into the lumen.[5]

However, accumulating potassium within principal cells does not necessarily strongly promote potassium secretion. The apical membrane pathways (see Figure 8–1) that allow potassium to exit the cell must be open. This is the function of the second important factor influencing potassium secretion by the principal cells, the hormone aldosterone, which, besides stimulating sodium reabsorption by the principal cells (Chapter 7), simultaneously enhances potassium secretion by activating apical potassium channels in principal cells (called ROMK because they were K channels first isolated from the *r*enal *o*uter *m*edulla, but now isoforms have been described in several other parts of the kidney). In addition, aldosterone stimulates the activity of basolateral membrane Na-K-ATPase pumps. This latter effect additionally increases basolateral potassium transport into the cell (above that driven by increased plasma potassium), hence increasing intracellular potassium concentration and the gradient for movement into the lumen.

The signaling pathway by which changes in plasma potassium produce changes in circulating levels of aldosterone is much more straightforward than the mechanisms by which changes in plasma volume control aldosterone production. Responses to plasma volume, as discussed in Chapter 7, involve the renin-angiotensin system, which stimulates the adrenal cortex; however, the aldosterone-secreting cells of the adrenal cortex are also sensitive to the potassium concentration of the ECF bathing them (Figure 8–2). Increased intake of potassium leads to increased extracellular potassium concentration, which, in turn, directly stimulates aldosterone production by the adrenal cortex. The resulting increase in plasma aldosterone concentration stimulates potassium channels in principal cells.

Aldosterone plays an additional role in potassium secretion. Although it might appear that stimulation of Na-K-ATPase and stimulation of potassium channels in principal cells should be sufficient to promote potassium secretion, a third factor is also important: the delivery of sodium to the cortical collecting duct. Recall from Chapter 7 that aldosterone increases the activity or number of luminal membrane sodium channels. Principal cells take up sodium through these sodium channels in the luminal membrane and pump the sodium into the cortical interstitium via the Na-K-ATPase. Potassium secretion is absolutely dependent on this process primarily because potassium cannot be taken up unless sodium is being pumped out by the Na-K-ATPase. With an increased delivery of sodium to the cortical collecting duct, more sodium enters principal cells, and more potassium

---

[5] Whether the variable uptake by principal cells is a direct effect of basolateral potassium concentration or the result of an unidentified signaling process is not clear.

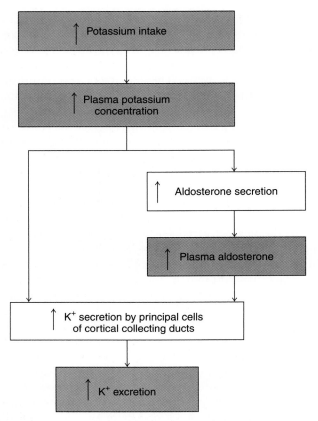

Figure 8–2. Pathways by which an increased potassium intake induces increased potassium excretion by increasing the potassium secretion by principal cells in the cortical collecting duct.

is secreted.[6] To some extent, the principal cells are exchanging one cation for another, moving luminal sodium into the cell and replacing it with cellular potassium that moves out of the cell into the lumen.

In contrast to the prior discussion that considered excess total-body potassium, below-normal extracellular potassium concentration tends to reverse all of the processes described previously. That is, a low-potassium diet or negative-potassium balance (eg, from diarrhea) lowers potassium concentration in the interstitium outside the principal cells and reduces Na-K-ATPase driven entry of potassium into principle cells. In addition, decreased potassium decreases aldosterone production, which reduces

---

[6] Another influence of sodium delivery is the effect on the apical membrane potential. A high sodium concentration in the lumen tends to depolarize the apical membrane, and this increases the passive driving force for potassium secretion.

potassium and sodium permeability of the apical membrane of principal cells, thereby reducing tubular potassium secretion. Less potassium than usual is excreted in the urine, thus helping to preserve the normal extracellular potassium concentration.

The examples used here have been concerned with changes in dietary potassium intake. However, it should be emphasized that when total-body potassium balance is perturbed by primary changes in potassium *output* (eg, in severe diarrhea), the same mechanisms described previously operate to control potassium secretion in the cortical collecting duct, thereby helping to restore potassium balance. Thus, potassium depletion resulting from diarrhea would tend to inhibit aldosterone secretion and, hence, potassium excretion. (The phrase "tend to inhibit" highlights the fact that, as we have seen, potassium is not the major regulator of aldosterone secretion; Figure 8–3.)

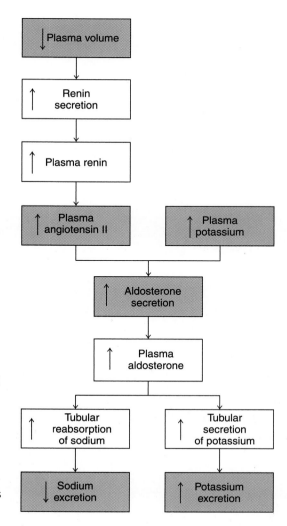

Figure 8–3. Summary of control of aldosterone by plasma volume and plasma potassium concentration and the effects of aldosterone on renal handling of sodium and potassium. Aldosterone also exerts a third effect on the tubule: It stimulates tubular hydrogen ion secretion, as described in Chapter 9.

It should be evident that a conflict will arise if decreases or increases in both potassium and plasma volume occur simultaneously, because these 2 changes drive aldosterone production in opposite directions. Whether aldosterone increases or decreases in such situations depends on the relative magnitudes of the opposing inputs. In general, changes in sodium balance and blood pressure have greater effects on aldosterone secretion than do equivalent changes in potassium balance.

This raises a potential problem for potassium homeostasis: If aldosterone secretion is altered via the renin-angiotensin system because of altered sodium balance, will the change in plasma aldosterone cause an imbalance of body potassium by inducing inappropriate changes in potassium secretion? In most physiological situations, the answer is no. Consider the following example (Figure 8–4). A person on a high-sodium diet has a low plasma aldosterone concentration because of elevated blood pressure and decreased renin secretion, and the reduced aldosterone will tend to decrease potassium

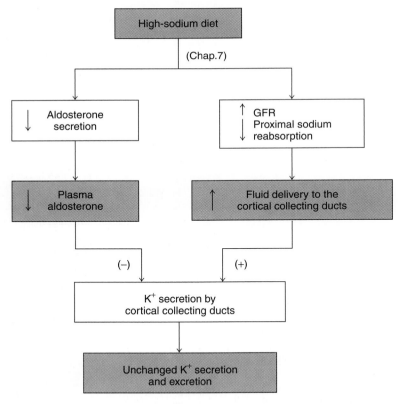

Figure 8–4. A high-sodium diet decreases plasma aldosterone (via the renin-angiotensin system) but simultaneously increases fluid delivery to the cortical collecting duct. These inputs have opposing effects on potassium secretion by the principal cells of the cortical collecting duct, so that little change occurs. GFR, glomerular filtration rate.

secretion. Simultaneously, however, the person on the high-sodium diet has both increased glomerular filtration rate and reduced proximal sodium reabsorption (because of reductions in renal interstitial hydraulic pressure, angiotensin II, and renal sympathetic input (Chapter 7), resulting in increased fluid delivery to the more distal tubular segments. The increased fluid flow through the cortical collecting duct tends to increase potassium secretion. The net result is that the effects on potassium secretion of the low aldosterone and high fluid delivery essentially counterbalance each other, and little if any change in potassium secretion and, hence, excretion occurs. Thus, the decreased aldosterone caused by increased sodium intake can increase sodium excretion without producing significant potassium retention.

Why should an increase in flow increase potassium secretion? The flow-induced increase in potassium secretion depends on the fact that movement of potassium across the apical membrane of principal cells is through an ion channel. Ion movement through channels is driven by concentration gradients (and potential). Increased luminal flow prevents accumulation of potassium and maintains a very low luminal concentration, thereby promoting secretion. This same explanation in reverse applies to sodium-depleted individuals and to those with congestive heart failure or other diseases of secondary hyperaldosteronism. Such persons have high aldosterone, which will tend to increase potassium secretion, but also low fluid delivery to the cortical collecting duct, which will tend to reduce potassium secretion. The net effect is relatively unchanged potassium secretion and excretion.

To summarize, changes in aldosterone secretion in either direction caused by changes in sodium balance do not usually cause major perturbations in potassium balance. This is because changes in sodium balance that lead to changes in aldosterone are usually associated with changes in *flow* through the cortical collecting duct, which counteracts the effect of the altered aldosterone on potassium secretion.

Effects of Diuretics

Diuretics are agents that increase urine volume and reduce ECF volume. Most diuretics, although effective at their designated task of increasing water and sodium excretion, have the unwanted side effect of increasing the renal excretion of potassium. Potassium excretion is almost always increased in individuals undergoing osmotic diuresis (high filtration of solute that is not reabsorbed) or treatment with diuretics that block sodium reabsorption in the proximal tubule, loop of Henle, or distal convoluted tubule (ie, block of sodium reabsorption upstream from the principal cells). The potassium loss may cause severe potassium depletion.

The increased potassium excretion is due partly to the fact that, as noted earlier, potassium reabsorption in the proximal tubule and Henle's loop is linked to sodium reabsorption. Accordingly, diuretics that act on these sites inhibit not only sodium reabsorption but also potassium reabsorption. However, *most* of the increased potassium excretion is due not to this decreased reabsorption but rather to increased potassium *secretion* by the cortical collecting duct. In all these diuretic states, the delivery of sodium and volume of fluid flowing into the collecting duct per unit time is increased by the upstream inhibition of sodium and water reabsorption. It is this

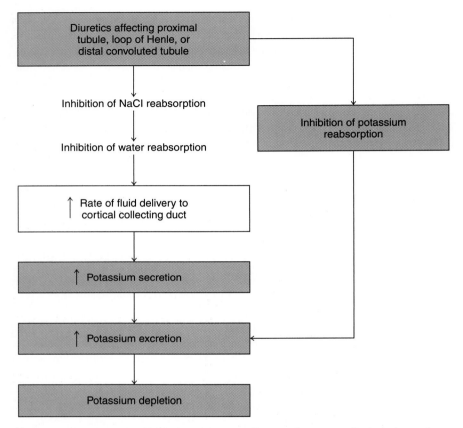

Figure 8–5. Pathway by which diuretic drugs affecting the proximal tubule, loop of Henle, or distal convoluted tubule cause potassium depletion. The decrease in potassium reabsorption is a less important factor in causing the increased potassium excretion than the increased secretion by the principal cells of the cortical collecting ducts.

increased flow and increased delivery of sodium that drives increased potassium secretion and, hence, excretion (Figure 8–5).

To reinforce this point further, let us integrate this information with our understanding of the action of aldosterone. Elevated aldosterone in individuals with heart failure or other diseases of secondary hyperaldosteronism generally does not cause potassium hypersecretion because these patients simultaneously have low fluid delivery to the cortical collecting duct. However, what happens when such persons are treated with diuretics to eliminate their retained sodium and water? The diuretics increase fluid delivery to the cortical collecting ducts, and now the patients have both increased aldosterone and increased flow to the cortical collecting duct. This combination tends to cause marked increases in potassium secretion and excretion. To prevent this combination, drugs that block the renal actions of aldosterone may be given; such drugs are weak diuretics because they block aldosterone's stimulation of sodium reabsorption (with its small amount of associated water reabsorption). However, unlike other diuretics, they are "potassium sparing" because they simultaneously block aldosterone's stimulation of potassium channels that promote potassium secretion. Another class of "potassium-sparing" diuretics blocks sodium channels in the principal cells of the cortical collecting duct; this prevents sodium entry from lumen to cell and effectively prevents the basolateral membrane Na-K-ATPase pumps from transporting either sodium or potassium and blocks the apical exchange of sodium for potassium ions. Blocking sodium absorption upstream from the cortical collecting duct increases potassium secretion; however, blocking sodium reabsorption *in the cortical collecting duct* does not.

Effects of Acid-Base Changes on Potassium Excretion

Primary acid-base disturbances are a major cause of secondary potassium imbalances (and, as discussed in Chapter 9, imbalances in body potassium can perturb acid-base status). These topics are fraught with difficulty because the effects are not consistently seen. Nevertheless, the existence of an elevated plasma pH (alkalosis) is often (ie, frequently but not always) associated with hypokalemia (low plasma potassium concentration). Similarly, low plasma pH (acidosis) is usually associated with hyperkalemia. Whether these relations between acid-base and potassium are actually seen in a particular patient depends on many factors, including the cause of the acid-base disturbance.

There are 2 known reasons for the effects of acid-base status on potassium. First, elevations and depressions in the extracellular concentration of hydrogen ions lead to a de facto exchange of these ions with cellular cations, the most important of which is potassium. During an alkalosis, for example, the low extracellular hydrogen ion concentration induces the efflux of hydrogen ions that are normally bound to cytosolic buffers. The loss of these cations is balanced by the uptake of other cations, in this case potassium. Thus, an alkalosis (with hydrogen ions leaving tissue cells to replenish the loss from the ECF) induces cells to take up potassium, causing a hypokalemia. Conversely, a low pH (with a concomitant cellular uptake of hydrogen ions) often leads cells to dump potassium, causing a hyperkalemia. Second, there is an effect of intracellular pH on cellular Na-K-ATPase and potassium channel activity. Low intracellular pH inhibits pumps everywhere, allowing potassium to escape from cells (particularly muscle cells) to increase plasma potassium. Ordinarily, the increase in plasma potassium would stimulate potassium uptake by the Na-K-ATPase in principal cells, but low intracellular pH also inhibits the pump here as well as luminal membrane potassium channels. Therefore, the principal cells respond inappropriately and do not effectively secrete the excess plasma potassium (*paradoxical potassium retention*). A high intracellular pH reverses these effects and relieves this inhibition (effectively stimulating the pump and the potassium channels). Alkalosis promotes potassium loss and contributes to the production of a hypokalemia. Thus, a patient suffering from alkalosis (induced, eg, by vomiting) will manifest increased urinary excretion of potassium solely as a result of the alkalosis and will, therefore, become potassium deficient.

Conversely, an acidosis *may* cause potassium retention. However, this phenomenon is seen less often than the potassium loss associated with alkalosis. Again, it should be emphasized that, although alkalosis is often associated with hypokalemia and acidosis with hyperkalemia, this is not always the case.

KEY CONCEPTS

 Only a small fraction of body potassium is extracellular, and the extracellular concentration may not be a good indicator of total-body potassium status.

 On a short-term basis, uptake and release of potassium by tissue cells prevent large swings in extracellular potassium concentration.

 Overall renal handling is accomplished by reabsorbing nearly all filtered potassium and then secreting an amount of potassium that maintains balance between ingestion and excretion.

 It is mainly the principal cells of the cortical collecting duct that alter rates of potassium secretion.

 Potassium secretion (and thus excretion) is increased by high sodium delivery to the distal nephron, particularly when this is caused by diuretics acting upstream.

 STUDY QUESTIONS

8–1. Control of potassium excretion is achieved mainly by regulating the rate of which of the following?
    A. Potassium filtration
    B. Potassium reabsorption
    C. Potassium secretion

8–2. When on a high-potassium or high-sodium diet, is it possible to excrete more potassium or sodium in the urine than is filtered?

8–3. Indicate whether each statement is true or false.
    A. In the proximal tubule, the major pathway of reabsorption for both sodium and potassium is paracellular.
    B. In the thick ascending limb, the major pathway of reabsorption for both sodium and potassium is via the Na-K-2Cl multiporter.
    C. In the thick ascending limb, equal amounts of sodium and potassium are absorbed.

8–4.   The presence of high amounts of nonreabsorbed solute (eg, glucose) in the proximal tubule inhibits proximal tubule potassium reabsorption. True or false?

8–5.   The presence of high amounts of nonreabsorbed solute (eg, glucose) in the collecting tubule inhibits potassium secretion. True or false?

8–6.   A patient has a tumor in the adrenal gland that continuously secretes large quantities of aldosterone (primary hyperaldosteronism). Is the rate of potassium excretion normal, high, or low?

8–7.   A patient with severe congestive heart failure is secreting large quantities of aldosterone. Is the rate of potassium excretion normal, high, or low?

Regulation of Hydrogen Ion Balance

9

OBJECTIVES

The student understands the interrelation among (1) input and output of acids and bases, (2) regulation of plasma buffers, and (3) value of plasma pH:

▶ *States the major sources for the input of fixed acids and bases into the body, including metabolic processes and activities of the gastrointestinal tract.*

▶ *Describes why carbon dioxide levels affect the concentration of hydrogen ions, and differentiates carbon dioxide input (volatile acid) from the input of fixed acids.*

▶ *States the Henderson-Hasselbalch equation for the carbon dioxide—bicarbonate buffer system.*

▶ *Describes how the input of fixed acids and bases affects the body levels of bicarbonate.*

▶ *Explains why body levels of carbon dioxide are usually not altered by the input of fixed acids and bases.*

▶ *Explains why some low pH fluids alkalinize the blood after they are metabolized.*

The student understands the general renal handling of acids and bases:

▶ *Describes the reabsorption of filtered bicarbonate by the proximal tubule, including the role of carbonic anhydrase and apical membrane Na-H antiporters.*

▶ *Describes how bicarbonate is excreted in response to an alkaline load.*

The student understands how the kidneys respond to an acid load:

▶ *Describes how excretion of acid and generation of new bicarbonate are linked.*

▶ *Defines the concept of urinary titratable acidity.*

▶ *Describes how the titration of filtered buffers is one means of excreting acid.*

▶ *Describes how the conversion of glutamine to ammonium and subsequent excretion of ammonium are equivalent to the excretion of acid.*

▶ *States how total acid excretion is related to titratable acidity and ammonium excretion.*

The student understands the nature of acid-base disturbances and the meaning of compensation:

▶ *Defines the 4 categories of primary acid-base disturbance.*

▶ *Defines the meaning of compensation.*

▶ *Describes the renal response to respiratory acid-base disorders.*

▶ *Describes the respiratory response to changes in arterial pH.*

▶ *Identifies nonrenal problems that may cause the kidneys to generate a metabolic alkalosis.*

GUIDELINES FOR STUDYING ACID-BASE BIOLOGY

The topic of acid-base physiology has vexed students for generations. Understanding acid-base physiology is greatly aided by keeping in mind several fundamental principles (outlined later) and always viewing its complexities through the lens of those fundamentals.

The essence of acid-base physiology is the operation of 2 sets of processes. The first is that the input and output of acids and bases from the body, obey the same principles of balance we have used in so many other aspects of renal function. The second is the regulation of the components of the main physiological buffer system, carbon dioxide (CO_2) and bicarbonate (HCO_3^-). In this buffer system the free concentration of hydrogen ions (or pH) is determined by the *ratio* of the blood concentrations of carbonic acid, the weak acid produced from CO_2 and water, and bicarbonate, carbonic acid's conjugate base. Balancing total-body input and output of acid or base and regulating physiological buffer concentrations are intimately related, but it is easy to lose sight of one perspective while seeing things from the other.

Guideline 1: Acids and Bases Obey the Balance Principle

Acids and bases are subject to the same constraints of input and output balance as other substances (eg, sodium, urea, and water). Each day, physiological processes add acids and bases to our body fluids, tending to raise or lower the concentration of hydrogen ions (change the pH). Each day, normal kidneys excrete acids and bases to exactly match the input, thereby keeping the body in acid-base balance. Despite the intricacies of acid-base balance, the basic principle of balance always holds. One reason to emphasize the balance concept is that, unlike substances such as sodium, there are multiple routes for the entry of acids or bases, including (1) de novo generation of acids and bases from metabolism, (2) activity of the gastrointestinal (GI) tract that adds acids or bases, and (3) processing of ingested food, which also adds acids or bases. Metabolism of stored fat and glycogen, depending on the metabolic pathways, can also add acid. In addition, of course, the kidneys are factors in the overall maintenance of hydrogen ion balance.

Another reason to emphasize the balance concept is to avert a common misconception about acid-base *disturbances,* situations in which either there is an unusually high input or output of acid or the plasma pH is abnormal (eg, diabetic ketoacidosis). Although the body is sometimes *transiently* out of balance for acids and bases (just as it is sometimes transiently out of balance for many other substances), acid-base disturbances do not mean there is a *persistent* imbalance. In a prolonged metabolic acidosis, for example, there may be a high input of acid and an equally high output. There is never a situation in which acid or base pours into the body for an extended period of time without being balanced by an equivalent output. However, being in acid-base balance (ie, the same input of acid as output) does not necessarily mean that there are no changes in body chemistry. As in the case for sodium balance, persistent excess sodium reabsorption does not continuously and indefinitely increase total-body sodium. Rather, other factors are stimulated to bring sodium back into balance, but the new balance state only comes at the price of elevated blood pressure. Input and output of hydrogen ion may be equal (in balance) during metabolic disorders that produce excess acid, but the balance comes about only after there has been a significant change in blood pH or bicarbonate concentration.

Guideline 2: Body Fluids Are Buffered

The most important buffer in the body is the CO_2–bicarbonate system. Consider what would happen if we did not have buffers. If we added strong acid (eg, hydrochloric acid) to water that contained no buffers, the concentration of protons would equal the concentration of the acid. If we had 10 mmol/L acid, we would have 10 mmol/L protons (ie, pH 2 blood). However, a buffered system contains weak acids, which only partially dissociate, and the conjugate base of those weak acids. In such a system, the free aqueous concentration of protons is only a trivial fraction of the concentration of the acid and is determined by the *ratio* of acid to its conjugate base. Simple mass action chemistry (Equation 9–1) describes how a weak acid dissociates into its conjugate base and a free hydrogen ion and how at equilibrium the concentration of free hydrogen ions is determined by the *ratio* of the concentrations of conjugate base to the weak acid (Equation 9–2) or in the more familiar pH form (the Henderson-Hasselbalch equation) in Equation 9–3.

A buffered system prevents large changes in pH after the addition or loss of protons from external sources. With the addition of hydrogen ions from an independent source (eg, food), most of the new hydrogen ions bind to the conjugate bases existing in the body fluids; only a small fraction of the added hydrogen ions remain free. In an analogous way, after removal of free hydrogen ions (eg, by addition of strong base), hydrogen ions are released from the existing weak acids, thus replacing most of those removed. The actions of a buffer system clamp the concentration of free hydrogen ions, and thus the pH, close to the original value.

Buffer systems do not have an infinite capacity to keep the concentration of hydrogen ions at a constant value because buffer is consumed in the reaction. However, they blunt the change in pH and give the kidneys time to alter their excretion and restore balance so that output again equals input.

$$\text{Acid} \leftrightarrow \text{conjugate base} + H^+ \tag{9–1}$$

$$[H] = K\,[\text{acid}]/[\text{base}] \tag{9–2}$$

$$pH = pK + \log[\text{base/acid}] \tag{9–3}$$

 What are the buffer systems in the body? Simply put, buffers exist in the extracellular fluid, the intracellular fluid (the cytosol of the various cells in the body), in the matrix of bone, and all of these systems communicate with each other.[1]

---

[1] Besides the crucial carbon dioxide–bicarbonate system, the ECF contains several other buffers that act in parallel; albumin and other plasma proteins have the largest capacity. ECF buffers react essentially instantaneously to an acid or base load. The intracellular fluid also contains buffers, more than the ECF, consisting of intracellular proteins and various phosphates that buffer acid and base loads on a time scale of hours. Hemoglobin in red blood cells is a key component, along with the enormous amount of protein in skeletal muscle. Buffering by bone is also significant (and rather complicated) on an even slower time scale.

As mentioned, quantitatively, the most important physiological buffer system is the CO_2–bicarbonate system. Unique features of the CO_2–bicarbonate buffer system make it different from other buffer systems. To understand physiological regulation of systemic pH, we must understand these differences. First, carbon dioxide is not an acid per se (it cannot donate a hydrogen ion by itself), but it reacts with water to form carbonic acid, and carbonic acid, as does any weak acid, partially dissociates into a hydrogen ion and a conjugate base (bicarbonate), as described in Equation 9–4. Most of the time, these species are in equilibrium.

The concentration of carbonic acid in our blood is miniscule (about 3 μmol/L), and at first glance it appears that this system has little effective buffering capacity. However, the supply of CO_2 is effectively infinite, so that any carbonic acid consumed in a reaction is replaced by new generation from existing CO_2.

$$CO_2 + H_2O \leftrightarrow H_2CO_3 \leftrightarrow HCO_3^- + H^+ \qquad (9\text{--}4)$$

The carbonic acid reaction on the left side of Equation 9–4 is rather slow, but most tissues express one or several isoforms of the enzyme, carbonic anhydrase, intracellularly, extracellularly, or both. This is an enzyme that greatly speeds the reaction to form bicarbonate and a hydrogen ion from CO_2 and water.[2] As with all enzyme catalyzed reactions, the enzyme increases the *velocity* of the reaction but does not change the equilibrium concentrations of reactants and products. On this basis, and given the ubiquitous presence of water in our body, it is clear that carbon dioxide is effectively an acid. Carbon dioxide is often called a *volatile* acid because it can escape from solution as a gas, in contrast to most other acids that are *fixed* acids (eg, lactic acid, sulfuric acid).

Guideline 3: Input and Output of Acids Alter Bicarbonate But Not Partial Pressure of CO_2

Unlike the other buffer systems in the body, where addition or loss of hydrogen ions changes the concentration of the weak acid, in the CO_2–bicarbonate system, the concentration of the weak acid (CO_2) is essentially constant. This is because the partial pressure of arterial CO_2 ($PaCO_2$) is regulated by our respiratory system to be about 40 mm Hg. This partial pressure corresponds to a CO_2 concentration in blood of 1.2 mmol/L. Any rise or fall in PCO_2 resulting from the addition or loss of hydrogen ions as depicted in Equation 9–4 is sensed by the respiratory centers in the brainstem that alter the rate of ventilation to restore the concentration. There are times when the PCO_2 differs from 40 mm Hg, but this reflects activity of the respiratory system, not a change in PCO_2 in response to addition or loss of hydrogen ions.

---

[2] The actual reaction involves combining CO_2 with a hydroxyl ion already bound to the enzyme, resulting in the immediate formation of bicarbonate (HCO_3^-). As the bicarbonate dissociates from the enzyme, a water molecule binds to it. The water is then split into a hydrogen ion that dissociates from the enzyme and a hydroxyl ion that stays behind on the enzyme. The end result is that a CO_2 molecule and a water molecule have been converted to a hydrogen ion and a bicarbonate, the same as if they had gone through the slower uncatalyzed reaction of first forming a carbonic acid molecule.

Although adding or removing hydrogen ions from an independent source (ie, a source other than CO_2) does not change P_{CO_2}, such changes *do* change the concentration of *bicarbonate*. Adding hydrogen ions drives the reaction in Equation 9-4 to the left and reduces bicarbonate on a nearly mole-for-mole basis. Removing hydrogen ions drives the reaction to the right and raises bicarbonate in the same way. There are many ways of adding or removing hydrogen ions, but, regardless of the process, the result is to change the concentration of bicarbonate. In summary, adding hydrogen ions reduces bicarbonate; removing hydrogen ions raises bicarbonate.

When any process puts hydrogen ions into the blood, most of the hydrogen ions, as we have emphasized, combine with the conjugate base of buffers, in this case bicarbonate. Now a protonated bicarbonate is simply a molecule of carbonic acid. When the concentration of carbonic acid rises, the carbonic acid dissociates into CO_2 and water. The CO_2 formed in this manner mixes with metabolic CO_2 and is exhaled, thus restoring the concentration of CO_2 and carbonic acid, but some bicarbonate has been lost. So when we add hydrogen ions by diet or some physiological process, we lose some bicarbonate but we do not change the P_{CO_2} or concentration of carbonic acid. Suppose we *remove* hydrogen ions. CO_2 and water combine to generate a hydrogen ion (replacing the one lost) and a bicarbonate. The CO_2 is supplied from the enormous store of metabolic CO_2. The P_{CO_2} remains constant (if it starts to change, ventilation adjusts to restore it). We end up with a gain in bicarbonate and no change in P_{CO_2}. Thus, addition or removal of hydrogen ion alters total-body bicarbonate; therefore, the problem of maintaining hydrogen ion balance becomes one of maintaining bicarbonate balance. For every hydrogen ion added to the body, one bicarbonate disappears; therefore, to maintain balance it is necessary to generate a new bicarbonate to replace the one that was lost. Generation of new bicarbonate is the responsibility of the kidney.

We have established that CO_2 is effectively an acid. Let us be sure we understand why normal metabolic production of CO_2 does not keep acidifying the body. An enormous of amount of CO_2 is generated from metabolism each day. It is produced in our body at a rate of about 9 mmol/min. However, it is *eliminated* at the same rate, so there is no *net* addition. On entering the blood flowing into tissue capillaries (arterial blood), the majority of the CO_2 immediately combines with water to form hydrogen ions and bicarbonate. Most of the hydrogen ions then combine with non-bicarbonate buffers (eg, hemoglobin), so the change in pH is not great, although there is a small drop in pH. The concentration of bicarbonate rises by about 1 mmol/L (from 24 to 25 mmol/L). When this blood carrying the newly loaded CO_2 (now venous blood) reaches the capillaries of the lungs, the processes that occurred in the tissue capillaries are reversed. Bicarbonate and hydrogen ions combine to generate CO_2 and water, and the CO_2 diffuses into the air spaces of the lungs. The pH rises a little, and the concentration of bicarbonate falls by about 1 mmol/L (back to 24 mmol/L).

Guideline 4: Excretion of CO_2 and Bicarbonate Are Independent of Each Other

Another situation that confuses students, and one that we also want to clarify immediately, is that the input and output of CO_2 and bicarbonate are handled *independently*:

One cannot be excreted as the other. If there is an excess generation of CO_2 (eg, if there is a rise in metabolism not matched by an increase in ventilation), the CO_2 cannot be converted to fixed acid and excreted by the kidneys. Increased CO_2 input must be balanced by increased CO_2 exhalation from the lungs. Similarly, if there is excess input of fixed acid (resulting in a lowering of bicarbonate), the body cannot convert this acid to CO_2 and excrete it through the lungs. This new input of fixed acid must be balanced by renal output.

Sources of Fixed Acids and Bases

METABOLISM OF DIETARY PROTEIN

Although the oxidative metabolism of most foodstuff is acid-base neutral, protein contains some amino acids that contribute acid or base. When sulfur- (or phosphorus-) containing amino acids and those with cationic side chains are metabolized to CO_2, water, and urea, the end result is addition of fixed acid. Similarly, the oxidative metabolism of amino acids with anionic side chains adds base (consumes hydrogen ions). Depending on whether a person's diet is high in meat or fruit and vegetables, the net input can be acid or base. For typical American diets the input is acidic.

METABOLISM OF DIETARY WEAK ACIDS

Fruits and vegetables, particularly citrus fruit, contain a lot of weak acids and the salts of those acids (ie, the conjugate base plus a cation, usually potassium). We all know that citrus fruit is acidic, with some fruit juices having a pH below 4.0. Interestingly, metabolism of these acidic substances *alkalinizes* the blood, sometimes called the *fruit juice paradox*. The complete oxidation of the protonated form of an organic acid (eg, citric acid) to CO_2 and water is acid-base neutral, no different in principle than the oxidation of glucose. However, the complete oxidation of the base form adds bicarbonate to the body. One can think of this as taking a hydrogen ion from the body fluids to protonate the base, converting it to the acid, and then oxidizing the acid. Acidic fruits and vegetables contain a mixture of organic acids in the protonated form and base form. Before oxidation, the mixture is acidic, but on complete oxidation to CO_2 and water, the result is addition of base.

GI SECRETIONS

The GI tract, from the salivary glands to the colon, is lined with an epithelium that can secrete hydrogen ions, bicarbonate, or a combination. In addition, the major exocrine secretions of the pancreas and liver that flow into the duodenum contain large amounts of bicarbonate. Normally, the sum of these secretions is nearly acid-base neutral (ie, the secretion of acid in one site, eg, the stomach) is balanced by the secretion of bicarbonate elsewhere (eg, the pancreas). However, in conditions of vomiting or diarrhea, one kind of secretion may dominate. It is important to note (Figure 9–1) that secretion of hydrogen ions across the apical membrane of an epithelial cell into a lumen (GI tract or nephron) is always accompanied by the transport of a bicarbonate across the basolateral membrane into the surrounding interstitium (and then into the blood). That is, GI secretion of hydrogen ions puts base

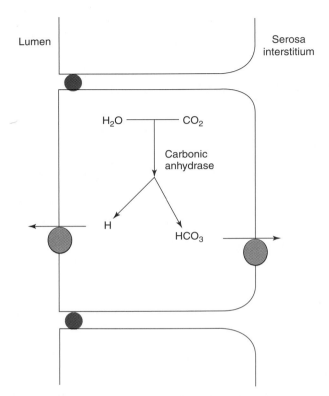

Figure 9–1. Generic model for the secretion of hydrogen ions. The source of secreted hydrogen ions is CO_2 and water. Every secreted hydrogen ion must be accompanied by the transport of a bicarbonate into the interstitium.

(bicarbonate) into the blood. Similarly, the secretion of bicarbonate into the GI tract puts hydrogen ions into the blood.

ANAEROBIC METABOLISM OF CARBOHYDRATE AND FAT

The normal oxidative metabolism of carbohydrate and fat is acid-base neutral. Both carbohydrate (glucose) and triglycerides are oxidized to CO_2 and water. Although there are intermediates in the metabolism (eg, pyruvate) that are acids or bases, the sum of all the reactions is neutral. However, some conditions lead to production of fixed acids. The anaerobic metabolism of carbohydrate produces a fixed acid (lactic acid). In conditions of poor tissue perfusion, this can be a major acidifying factor, and the metabolism of triglyceride to β-hydroxybutyrate and acetoacetate also adds fixed acid (ketone bodies). These processes normally do not add much of an acid load but can add a huge acid load in unusual metabolic conditions (eg, diabetes).

There are other ways of adding acids or bases (eg, by ingestion of certain drugs or other foreign materials and by intravenous infusions). However, there is typically a small net load of acid or base resulting from normal metabolism of foodstuff and from GI processes. This load can be greatly increased in unusual circumstances. If the kidneys are working properly, they excrete the load, small or large, and keep the body in balance.

RENAL HANDLING OF ACIDS AND BASES

A simplified overview of the renal processing of acids and bases is as follows: In the early part of the nephron (mostly proximal tubule), the kidneys reabsorb the enormous filtered load of bicarbonate (thereby resulting in no addition or loss) and, under appropriate conditions, can secrete organic bases or weak organic acids and acid equivalents. Then, in the distal nephron (mostly the collecting tubules), the kidneys secrete either protons or bicarbonate to balance the net input into the body (summarized in Table 9–1).

The first task is to reabsorb filtered bicarbonate. Bicarbonate is freely filtered at the renal corpuscles. How much is normally filtered per day? Given a typical plasma concentration of 24 mmol/L and a glomerular filtration rate (GFR) of 180 L/day, this amounts to 4320 mmol/day. Excretion of this bicarbonate would be equivalent to adding more than 4 L of 1 N acid to the body! It is essential, therefore, that virtually all the filtered bicarbonate be reabsorbed or the body fluids would become profoundly acidic. Thus, the reabsorption of bicarbonate is an essential conservation process.

Bicarbonate reabsorption is an active process, but it is not accomplished in the conventional manner simply through an active transporter for bicarbonate ions at either the luminal or basolateral membrane. Rather, the mechanism by which bicarbonate is reabsorbed involves the tubular secretion of hydrogen ions.

An enormous amount of hydrogen ion secretion occurs in the proximal tubule, with additional secretion in the thick ascending limb of Henle's loop and collecting-duct system. In contrast to the situation for handling sodium, water, and potassium, the collecting-duct cells that secrete hydrogen ion are the Type A intercalated cells, not the principal cells.

Table 9–1. Normal contributions of tubular segments to renal hydrogen ion balance

Proximal tubule
  Reabsorbs most filtered bicarbonate (normally about 80%)*
  Produces and secretes ammonium

Thick ascending limb of Henle's loop
  Reabsorbs second largest fraction of filtered bicarbonate (normally about 10–15%)*

Distal convoluted tubule and collecting-duct system
  Reabsorbs virtually all remaining filtered bicarbonate as well as any secreted bicarbonate
    (Type A intercalated cells)*
  Produces titratable acid (Type A intercalated cells)*
  Secretes bicarbonate (Type B intercalated cells)

* Processes achieved by hydrogen ion secretion.

The basic pattern followed in all these tubular segments is the same (although the precise transporters involved differ to some extent) and is illustrated in Figure 9–1 without indicating any specific transporters. Within the cells, a hydrogen ion and a bicarbonate are generated from CO_2 and water, catalyzed by carbonic anhydrase. The hydrogen ion is actively secreted into the tubular lumen. For every hydrogen ion secreted, 1 bicarbonate ion is generated within the cell. The bicarbonate is transported across the basolateral membrane into the interstitial fluid and then into the peritubular capillary blood. The net result is that, for every hydrogen ion secreted into the lumen, a bicarbonate ion enters the blood in the peritubular capillaries. There must be a 1-for-1 match between hydrogen ions secreted and bicarbonate ions transported into the interstitium.

The source of secreted hydrogen ions is CO_2 and water; therefore, the rate of hydrogen ion secretion is exactly matched by the intracellular production of bicarbonate. What is the fate of this bicarbonate? Clearly, the bicarbonate cannot just accumulate; otherwise, our kidney cells would turn into clumps of baking soda. It cannot be neutralized by a hydrogen ion because the only source of hydrogen ions is the very process that generates the bicarbonate. The bicarbonate could theoretically be secreted in parallel with the hydrogen ions, but this would be a useless process; the hydrogen ions and bicarbonate would just combine in the lumen. Therefore, the only useful fate for bicarbonate is to be transported across the basolateral membrane.

Specific transporters are required for the transmembrane movements of both the hydrogen ion and the bicarbonate. Active transport of hydrogen ion across the luminal membrane from cell to lumen is achieved by several distinct luminal membrane transporters. First, particularly prominent in the proximal tubule is an Na-H antiporter as described in Chapter 6 (Figure 9–2). This transporter is the major means not only of hydrogen ion secretion but also of sodium uptake from the proximal tubule lumen. Second, a primary active H-ATPase exists in all the hydrogen ion-secreting distal tubular segments. The Type A intercalated cells of the collecting-duct system, in addition to their primary active H-ATPase, possess a primary active H-K-ATPase, which simultaneously moves hydrogen ions into the lumen and potassium into the cell, both actively (Figure 9–3). Note that, as described in Chapter 8, the luminal membrane H-K-ATPase also mediates active potassium reabsorption by these cells.

The basolateral membrane exit step for bicarbonate is via $Cl-HCO_3$ antiporters or $Na-HCO_3$ symporters (see Figure 9–2), depending on the tubular segment. In both cases, the movement of bicarbonate is down its electrochemical gradient (ie, the transport is passive). The symport with sodium is particularly interesting because efflux of sodium is *up* its electrochemical gradient. This is a rare case of sodium active transport not using an Na-K-ATPase.[3]

Figure 9–4 illustrates how the process of hydrogen ion secretion (Figure 9–1) achieves bicarbonate reabsorption. Once in the tubular lumen, a secreted hydrogen ion combines with a *filtered* bicarbonate to form water and carbon dioxide, which diffuse into the cell (and can be used by the cell in another cycle). The overall result is

---

[3] Ultimately, the process requires the activity of the Na-K-ATPase. This transporter is needed to maintain a low enough intracellular sodium concentration so that the apical membrane Na-H antiporter will secrete hydrogen ions.

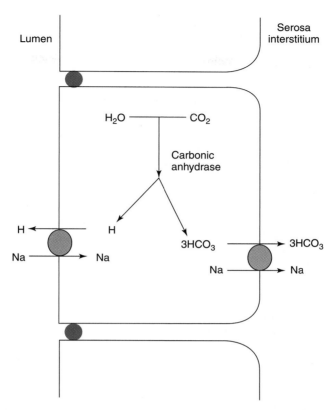

Figure 9–2. Predominant proximal tubule mechanism for the secretion of hydrogen ions that result in reabsorption of bicarbonate. Hydrogen ions are secreted via an Na-H antiporter (member of the NHE family). Bicarbonate is transported into the interstitium via an Na-HCO$_3$ symporter (member of the NBC family).

that the bicarbonate filtered from the blood at the renal corpuscle has disappeared, but its place in the blood has been taken by the bicarbonate that was produced inside the cell. Thus, no net change in plasma bicarbonate concentration has occurred. It may seem inaccurate to refer to this process as bicarbonate reabsorption because the bicarbonate that appears in the peritubular capillary is not the same bicarbonate that was filtered. Yet the overall result is the same as it would be if the filtered bicarbonate had been more conventionally reabsorbed, like a sodium or potassium ion.

It is also important to note that the hydrogen ion that was secreted into the lumen is not excreted in the urine. It has been incorporated into water. Any secreted hydrogen ion that combines with bicarbonate in the lumen to cause bicarbonate reabsorption does not contribute to the urinary excretion of hydrogen ions but only to the conservation of bicarbonate.

Through its secretion of hydrogen ions, the proximal tubule reabsorbs 80–90% of the filtered bicarbonate. The thick ascending limb of Henle's loop reabsorbs

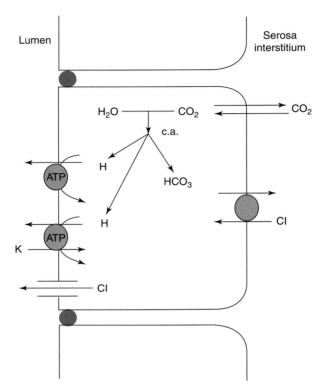

Figure 9–3. Predominant collecting tubule mechanisms in Type A intercalated cells for the secretion of hydrogen ions that result in formation of titratable acidity. The apical membrane contains H-ATPases that transport hydrogen ions alone or in exchange for potassium. c.a., carbonic anhydrase.

another 10%, and almost all the remaining bicarbonate is normally reabsorbed by the distal convoluted tubule and collecting-duct system (except for alkalotic individuals, who will excrete some of the bicarbonate; see later discussion).

Throughout the tubule, intracellular carbonic anhydrase is involved in the reactions generating hydrogen ion and bicarbonate. In the proximal tubule, carbonic anhydrase is also located in the lumen-facing surface of apical cell membranes, and this carbonic anhydrase catalyzes the intraluminal generation of CO_2 and water from the large quantities of secreted hydrogen ions combining with filtered bicarbonate.

Another important point needs to be made about bicarbonate reabsorption by the proximal tubule: There exists excellent glomerulotubular balance for bicarbonate reabsorption analogous to that described in Chapter 7 for sodium. When there is an increased filtered load of bicarbonate, whether caused by an increased GFR or an increased plasma bicarbonate concentration, the proximal tubule automatically reabsorbs more. The proximal tubule still reabsorbs approximately 80% of the filtered load,

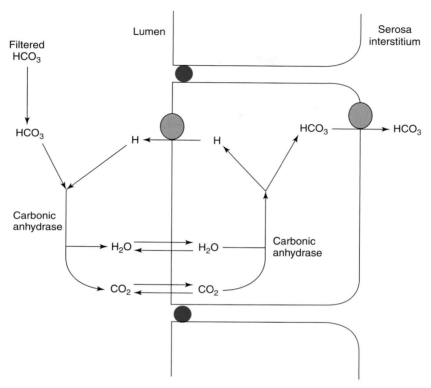

Figure 9–4. General mechanism for reabsorption of filtered bicarbonate. A secreted hydrogen ion combines with a filtered bicarbonate to form CO_2 and water in the lumen, catalyzed by extracellular carbonic anhydrase present in the cell brush border. The CO_2 and water formed in this process simply mix with the existing quantities of those substances. The bicarbonate generated intracellularly is transported into the interstitium and then back into peritubular capillaries. Because a filtered bicarbonate disappears and a new one is moved from cell to the blood, it is as though no bicarbonate had been filtered in the first place.

but the filtered load is larger. There must be a built-in mechanism for increasing proximal tubular hydrogen ion secretion when filtered load of bicarbonate increases. One simple mechanism is the decrease in free hydrogen ion concentration in the lumen of the proximal tubule when delivery of bicarbonate is increased. This decrease provides a natural driving force to increase the rate of the apical Na-H antiport.

RENAL EXCRETION OF ACID AND BASE

If all the filtered bicarbonate is reabsorbed, there is no acid-base consequence for the body; it is as though none had been filtered in the first place. When base has been added to the body fluids, the effect is to increase the plasma concentration of bicarbonate.

Whether this results from metabolism of protein that contains many anionic amino acids or from ingestion of baking soda (sodium bicarbonate), the result is the same: The body fluids contain more bicarbonate. The renal handling of base loads is relatively straightforward: We excrete some bicarbonate in the urine. If the addition of base to the body is 30 mEq and the kidneys put out 30 mmol of bicarbonate, the kidneys have achieved their goal: balance. The kidneys do this in 2 ways: (1) allow *some* filtered bicarbonate to pass through to the urine and (2) secrete bicarbonate via Type B intercalated cells. The Type B intercalated cells, which are found only in the cortical collecting duct, do indeed *secrete* bicarbonate. In essence, the Type B intercalated cell is a "flipped-around" Type A intercalated cell (Figure 9–5). Within the cytosol, hydrogen ions and bicarbonate are generated via carbonic anhydrase.

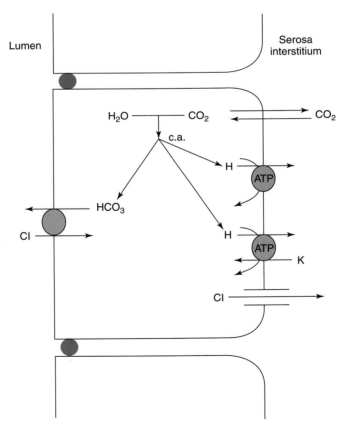

Figure 9–5. Type B intercalated cell. This cell type secretes bicarbonate and simultaneously transports hydrogen ions into the interstitium. The difference between this cell type and those shown earlier (that secrete hydrogen ions) is that the location of the transporters for hydrogen ions and bicarbonate are switched between apical and basolateral membranes. ATP, adenosine triphosphate; c.a., carbonic anhydrase.

However, the H-ATPase pump is located in the basolateral membrane, and the Cl-HCO_3 antiporter is in the luminal membrane. Accordingly, bicarbonate moves into the tubular lumen, whereas hydrogen ion is actively transported out of the cell across the basolateral membrane and enters the blood, where it can combine with a bicarbonate ion. Thus, the overall process achieves the disappearance of a plasma bicarbonate and the excretion of a bicarbonate in the urine, with resulting acidification of the plasma and alkalinization of the urine.

How do the kidneys excrete an *acid* load? For all individuals who ingest animal protein of any kind, removal of excess acid is more typical than the production and removal of excess base. This is a more complex process than excretion of base, but it obeys the principles we have developed earlier. Recall that the net result of addition of acid to the body reduces the amount of bicarbonate on an almost mole-for-mole basis. Therefore, the task for the kidney is to replace the lost bicarbonate by generating new bicarbonate from CO_2 and water (being careful to excrete the hydrogen ion that is created at the same time). The essence is as follows: Hydrogen ions are secreted and combine with the conjugate base of buffers *other than bicarbonate,* thereby generating the acid form of the buffer. The acid form of that buffer is excreted in the urine. The process of secreting hydrogen ions generates new bicarbonate that goes into the blood and neutralizes the acid load. The key is generation of *new* bicarbonate to replace the bicarbonate that was used up neutralizing hydrogen ions from ingested or metabolically produced fixed acids. If we just reabsorb filtered bicarbonate, nothing is changed. We must generate *new* bicarbonate.

HYDROGEN ION EXCRETION ON URINARY BUFFERS

We emphasized earlier how hydrogen ion secretion achieves bicarbonate reabsorption and how this process prevents loss of filtered bicarbonate. Now we see that the identical transport process of hydrogen ion secretion can also achieve acid excretion and addition of *new* bicarbonate to the blood. At first glance, this seems like a contradiction: How can the same process produce 2 different end results? The answers lies in the fate of the hydrogen ion once it is in the lumen. If the secreted hydrogen ion combines with bicarbonate, then we are simply replacing a bicarbonate that would have left the body. In contrast, if the secreted hydrogen ion combines with a *non-bicarbonate* buffer in the lumen (or, to an extremely small degree, remains free in solution), the hydrogen ion is excreted. The bicarbonate transported across the basolateral membrane is *new* bicarbonate, not a replacement for existing bicarbonate.

Normally, the most important of these filtered buffers is phosphate. Figure 9–6 illustrates the sequence of events that achieves hydrogen ion excretion on phosphate and the addition of new bicarbonate to the blood. The process of hydrogen ion secretion in this sequence is exactly the same as described previously, but the secreted hydrogen ion reacts in the lumen with filtered phosphate rather than with filtered bicarbonate. Therefore, the bicarbonate generated within the tubular cell (that always occurs when hydrogen ions are secreted) enters the plasma and constitutes a net gain of bicarbonate by the blood, not merely a replacement for a filtered bicarbonate. Thus, when a secreted hydrogen ion combines in the lumen with a filtered buffer other than bicarbonate, the

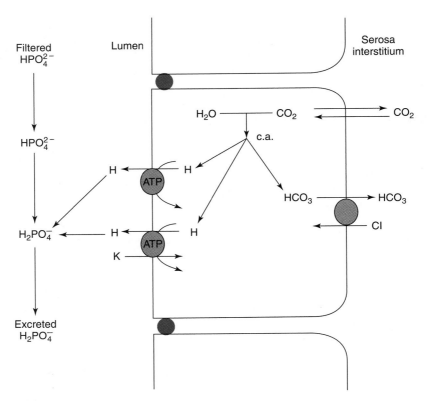

Figure 9–6. Excretion of hydrogen ions on filtered phosphate. Divalent phosphate (base form) that has been filtered and not reabsorbed reaches the collecting tubule, where it combines with secreted hydrogen ions to form monovalent phosphate (acid form) and is then excreted in the urine. The bicarbonate entering the blood is new bicarbonate, not merely a replacement for filtered bicarbonate. ATP, adenosine triphosphate; c.a., carbonic anhydrase.

overall effect is not merely bicarbonate conservation but rather addition to the blood of a new bicarbonate, which raises the bicarbonate concentration of the blood and the pH to a value similar to what it was before the addition of fixed acids.

Figure 9–6 also demonstrates another important point: namely, that the renal contribution of new bicarbonate to the blood is accompanied by the excretion of an equivalent amount of buffered hydrogen ion in the urine. In this case, in contrast to the reabsorption of bicarbonate, the secreted hydrogen ion remains in the tubular fluid, trapped there by the buffer, and is excreted in the urine. This should reinforce the concept that bicarbonate can always be generated from CO_2 and water, but to add this new bicarbonate to the blood (and alkalinize the blood), the kidneys must excrete from the body the hydrogen ion that is created at the same time.

It must be emphasized that neither *filtration* of hydrogen ions nor excretion of *free* hydrogen ions make a significant contribution to hydrogen ion excretion. First, the filtered load of free hydrogen ions, when the plasma pH is 7.4, is less than 0.1 mmol/day. Second, there is a minimum urinary pH—approximately 4.4—that can be achieved. This corresponds to a free hydrogen ion concentration of 0.04 mmol/L. With a typical daily urine output of 1.5 L, the excretion of *free* hydrogen ions is only 0.06 mmol/day, a tiny fraction of the normal 50–100 mmol ingested or produced every day.

PHOSPHATE AND ORGANIC ACIDS AS BUFFERS

Filtered phosphate is normally the most important non-bicarbonate urinary buffer. Most free plasma phosphate exists in a mixture of monovalent and divalent forms. In the following expression, monovalent phosphate (on the left) is a weak acid, and divalent phosphate (on the right) is its conjugate base.

$$H_2PO_4^- \leftrightarrow H^+ + HPO_4^{2-}$$

We can write this in the form of the Henderson-Hasselbalch equation:

$$pH = 6.8 + \log [HPO_4^{2-}]/[H_2PO_4^-]$$

At the normal pH of plasma (7.4) and, therefore, of the glomerular filtrate, we find that about 80% of the phosphate is in the base (divalent) form and 20% is in the acid (monovalent) form. As the tubular fluid is acidified in the collecting ducts, most of the secreted hydrogen ions combine with the base form. By the time the minimum intratubular pH of 4.4 is reached, virtually all of the base (HPO_4^{2-}) has been converted to acid ($H_2PO_4^-$). Therefore, secreted hydrogen ions that combined with the base form are excreted, and the bicarbonate that was generated intracellularly in the process enters the blood. How much phosphate is available for this process? The amount is quite variable, depending on a number of factors. A typical plasma concentration is about 1 mmol/L, of which about 90% is free (the rest being loosely bound to plasma proteins). At a GFR of 180 L/day, the filtered load of total phosphate is about 160 mmol/day. The fraction reabsorbed is also variable: from 75% to 90%. Thus, unreabsorbed divalent phosphate available for buffering is roughly 40 mmol/day. In other words, the kidneys can excrete hydrogen ions, using the phosphate buffer system, at rate of about 40 mmol/day.

There are other organic buffers in the urine, and under certain conditions these may appear in the tubular fluid in sufficient quantities to allow them also to act as important buffers. A particularly important example is the patient with uncontrolled diabetes mellitus. Because of metabolic processes that result from insulin deficiency, such a patient may become extremely acidotic because of so much production of acetoacetic acid and β-hydroxybutyric acid. At normal plasma pH, these species completely dissociate to yield the anions β-hydroxybutyrate and acetoacetate (and hydrogen ions). These anions are filtered at the renal corpuscle but are only partly reabsorbed because they are present in great enough quantities to exceed the renal reabsorptive T_ms for them. Accordingly, they are available in the tubular fluid to buffer a portion of the hydrogen ions being secreted by the tubules. However, their usefulness in this role is limited by the fact that their pKs are low: approximately 4.5. This means that only about half of these anions will be titrated by secreted hydrogen ions before the limiting urine pH of 4.4 is reached (ie, only half of them can actually be used as buffers).

HYDROGEN ION EXCRETION ON AMMONIUM

Ordinarily, hydrogen ion excretion associated with phosphate is about 40 mmol/day. This amount is not sufficient to balance the normal hydrogen ion production of 50 to 100 mmol/day. To excrete the rest of the hydrogen ion and achieve balance, there is a second means of excreting hydrogen ions that involves excretion of ammonium. Quantitatively, more hydrogen ions can be excreted by means of ammonium than organic buffers. There are many nuances to hydrogen ion excretion via ammonium, but the basic concepts are straightforward.

The catabolism of protein and oxidation of the constituent amino acids by the liver generates CO_2, water, urea, and some glutamine. Protein catabolism, which occurs constantly, even in starvation, requires the continuous excretion of urea by the kidneys to prevent uremia. Although, as described earlier, metabolism of the side chains of amino acids can lead to addition of acid or base, the processing of the core of an amino acid—the carboxyl group and amino group—is acid-base neutral. After many intermediate steps, processing of the carboxyl group of the amino acid produces a bicarbonate, and processing of the amino group produces an ammonium ion. Processing does not stop there, however, because ammonium in more than miniscule levels is quite toxic. Ammonium is further processed by the liver to urea or glutamine. In both cases, each ammonium consumed also consumes a bicarbonate. Thus, the bicarbonate produced from the carboxyl group is just an intermediate, consumed as fast as it is made, and does not add to body levels. We can write this process as follows:

$$2 \text{ amino acids (+oxygen)} \rightarrow 2NH_4^+ + 2HCO_3^- \rightarrow \text{urea or glutamine (+CO}_2 \text{ and water)}$$

When the urea (or glutamine) is excreted, the body has completed the catabolism of protein in a manner that is acid-base neutral.

Renal handling of urea is somewhat complicated from the osmotic point of view, as described in earlier chapters, but the handling is acid-base neutral. Glutamine, however, is different. Although the production of glutamine is acid-base neutral, it is important to recognize that glutamine can be thought to contain 2 components: a base component, bicarbonate, and an acid component, ammonium. Ammonium is an *extremely* weak acid (pK ~ 9.2), but an examination of the reversible reaction in which ammonium releases a hydrogen ion and the base (ammonia) demonstrates that ammonium is an acid nonetheless (because it is a hydrogen ion donor).

$$NH_4^+ \leftrightarrow H^+ + NH_3$$

Glutamine released from the liver is taken up by proximal tubule cells, both from the lumen (filtered glutamine) and from the renal interstitium. The cells of the proximal tubule then convert the glutamine back to bicarbonate and NH_4^+. In essence, the proximal tubule reverses what the liver has done. The NH_4^+ is secreted by the Na-H antiporter into the lumen of the proximal tubule,[4] and the bicarbonate exits into the interstitium and then into the blood (Figure 9–7). This is *new* bicarbonate, just like the new bicarbonate generated by titrating non-bicarbonate buffers. Further processing of the NH_4^+ is somewhat complex,[5] but eventually the ammonium is excreted (Figure 9–8).

A comparison of Figures 9–6 and 9–7 demonstrates that the overall result of renal generation of a new bicarbonate is the same regardless of whether it is achieved by hydrogen ion secretion and excretion on buffers (Figure 9–6) or by glutamine metabolism with NH_4^+ excretion (Figure 9–7 and 9–8). It is convenient, therefore, to view the latter case as representing H+ excretion in the form of an H+ "bound" to NH_3, just as the former case constitutes hydrogen ions bound to phosphate or other non-bicarbonate buffers. In this manner, we can, in both cases, quantitatively equate the terms *H+ excretion* and *renal contribution of new bicarbonate*.

QUANTIFICATION OF RENAL ACID-BASE EXCRETION

We can now quantify the kidneys' contribution to hydrogen ion balance. In other words, we can calculate the kidneys' net bicarbonate addition to the body or elimination from it. This value is, again, identical to the kidneys' net excretion of hydrogen ions ("acid"). Such a calculation is made by answering 3 questions:

1. How much bicarbonate is excreted in the urine? This represents bicarbonate loss from the body. It is measured simply by multiplying the urine flow rate by the urinary bicarbonate concentration.

2. How much new bicarbonate is contributed to the plasma by secretion of hydrogen ions that combine in the tubular lumen with non-bicarbonate urinary buffers? This can be measured by titrating the urine with NaOH to a pH of 7.4, the pH of the plasma from which the glomerular filtrate originated. This simply reverses the events that occurred within the tubular lumen when the tubular fluid was titrated by secreted hydrogen ions. Thus, the number of milliequivalents of sodium hydroxide required to reach pH 7.4 must equal the number of milliequivalents of hydrogen ion added to the tubular fluid that combined with phosphate and organic buffers. This value is known as the *titratable acid*.

3. How much new bicarbonate is returned to the plasma by secretion of hydrogen ions that are excreted as ammonium? The titratable acid measurement will not titrate hydrogen ions in NH_4^+ because ammonium is such a weak acid with

---

[4] Ammonium ion is interesting in that it can masquerade as other ions, in this case as a hydrogen ion and in other cases as a potassium ion. This is because some transporters and some channels are not completely selective for the species they usually move relative to ammonium.

[5] Ammonium entering the lumen in the proximal tubule is reabsorbed in the thick ascending limb, mostly by the NKCC multiporter, and accumulates in the medullary interstitium. This prevents the highly toxic ammonium ion from re-entering the renal cortex, where it would damage distal nephron epithelial cells. It is secreted again in the medullary collecting ducts. The medullary collecting ducts are permeable to ammonia so that ammonia diffuses into the lumen and combines with a secreted H+ to reform ammonium, which is impermeable. Therefore, the ammonium (with its associated hydrogen ion) is trapped in the lumen and is finally excreted.

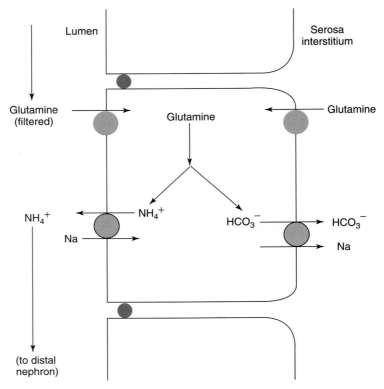

Figure 9–7. Ammonium production from glutamine. Glutamine is originally synthesized in the liver from NH_4^+ and bicarbonate. When it reaches the proximal tubule cells, it is converted back to NH_4^+ and bicarbonate. There are more biochemical steps in the conversion of glutamine to ammonium and bicarbonate than indicated here; only the end result is shown. The subsequent renal handling of ammonium involves reabsorption into the medullary interstitium of ammonium and subsequent secretion of ammonium from the interstitium into the collecting duct, where ultimately the ammonium generated from glutamine is excreted.

a pK of the ammonia-ammonium reaction so high (9.2) that titration with alkali to pH 7.4 will not remove hydrogen ions from NH_4^+.

Therefore, to know how much new bicarbonate is contributed by glutamine metabolism with ammonium excretion, urinary ammonium excretion (urine flow rate times urinary ammonium concentration) must be measured separately, remembering that for every ammonium excreted a new bicarbonate was added to the blood.

Thus, the data required for a quantitative assessment of the renal contribution to acid-base regulation in any person are as follows:

1. Titratable acid excreted
2. Plus NH_4^+ excreted

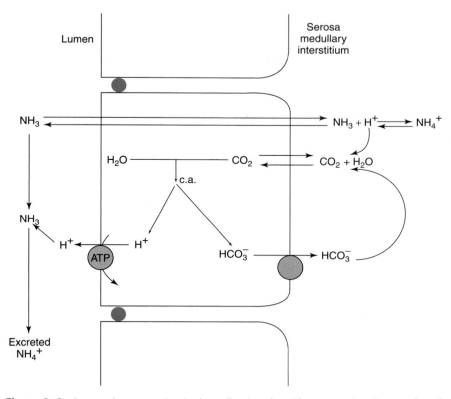

Figure 9–8. Ammonium excretion in the collecting duct. The ammonium ion produced from glutamine in the proximal tubule cells is reabsorbed in the thick ascending limb and enters the medullary interstitium. The medullary interstitium is impermeable to ammonium ion but not to ammonia (the dissociation product of ammonium). Ammonia is freely permeable through the epithelial cells and diffuses into the tubular lumen. Once in the lumen, it recombines with hydrogen ion secreted by hydrogen ATPases. Once the ammonia combines with hydrogen ion, the ammonium is trapped in the lumen and is excreted. This excretion of ammonium removes 1 hydrogen ion equivalent from the body. Because the original reaction that generated ammonium also generates a bicarbonate, the overall nephron handling of glutamine excretes 1 hydrogen ion and returns 1 bicarbonate to the blood. Because glutamine production can be stimulated by acidosis, the metabolism of glutamine and subsequent excretion of ammonium and return of bicarbonate to the blood is an effective way to counteract excessive ingestion or production of acids in the body. ATP, adenosine triphosphate; c.a., carbonic anhydrase.

3. Minus HCO_3^- excreted (ie, HCO_3^- lost from the body because of incomplete reabsorption or HCO_3^- secretion)

The total equals the net HCO_3^- gain or loss to the body (negative values equal loss, positive values equal gain).

Table 9–2. Renal contribution of new bicarbonate to the blood in different states

	Alkalosis	Normal state	Acidosis
Titratable acid (mmol/day)	0	20	40
plus NH$_4^+$ excreted (mmol/day)	0	40	160
minus HCO$_3^-$ excreted (mmol/day)	80	1	0
Total (mmol/day)	–80	59	200
	(*lost* from body)	(*added* to body)	(*added* to body)
Urine pH	8.0	6.0	4.6

Note that there is no term for free hydrogen ion in the urine because, even at a minimum urine pH of 4.4, the number of free hydrogen ions is trivial.

Typical urine data for the amounts of bicarbonate contributed to the blood by the kidneys in 3 potential acid-base states are given in Table 9–2. Note that in response to acidosis,[6] as emphasized previously, increased production and excretion of NH$_4^+$ is quantitatively much more important than increased formation of titratable acid.

It should also be emphasized that the data shown for alkalosis are typical of "pure" alkalosis (ie, alkalosis uncomplicated by other electrolyte abnormalities). As we will see, electrolyte imbalances frequently complicate alkalosis so that the expected values are different from those actually measured.

REGULATION OF THE RENAL HANDLING OF ACIDS AND BASES

It is clear that renal acid-base processing is regulated in response to different body conditions. Because a comprehensive description of how this occurs is beyond the scope of this text, we instead cover a few of the basic concepts.

When acid-base status is normal (Table 9–2), the tubules should secrete enough hydrogen ions to achieve essentially complete reabsorption of all filtered bicarbonate. Additional hydrogen ion will be secreted that will titrate buffers in the tubular lumen (titratable acid) and produce excreted ammonium, thereby returning new bicarbonate to the blood. (Recall that our diet usually produces net hydrogen ions that combine with bicarbonate to reduce total body bicarbonate. The amount of bicarbonate lost titrating hydrogen ion added to the blood must be generated by the kidneys to maintain balance.) During alkalosis, tubular secretion of hydrogen ion should be too low to completely reabsorb the filtered bicarbonate. Then bicarbonate can be lost in the urine; no titratable acid is formed because no extra secreted hydrogen ions are available to

---

[6] The suffixes "-osis" and "-emia" (meaning "in the blood"), as in acidosis or acidemia, are technically different but are often used interchangeably or inappropriately. Acidemia means high hydrogen ion concentration in the blood, essentially a pH below the normal range. Acidosis means a process adding acid to the blood. We can have an acidosis but not an acidemia if the pH is within the normal range and the kidneys are excreting the acid load as fast as it is added. The analogous argument applies to alkalemia and alkalosis. As will be seen, the proper distinction between "-osis" and "-emia" is violated in the common description of acid-base disorders.

combine with non-bicarbonate buffers, and so no new bicarbonate is contributed to the blood. During acidosis, tubular hydrogen ion secretion should be high enough to reabsorb all filtered bicarbonate and have enough hydrogen ions left to convert most of the base form of titratable buffers to the acid form, thereby contributing more new bicarbonate to the blood. (Recall, however, that this process is limited by the availability of buffers.) In addition, ammonium production should increase to excrete as ammonium the hydrogen ion that is not excreted as titratable acid. The production of ammonium also contributes new bicarbonate to the blood.

What, then, are the major homeostatic signals that influence tubular hydrogen ion secretion? They are Pa_{CO_2} and arterial pH. These signals act directly on the kidneys; no nerves or hormones are involved.

An increase in Pa_{CO_2}, as occurs during respiratory acidosis (eg, caused by shallow breathing after chest trauma),[7] causes an increased hydrogen ion secretion. A decrease in Pa_{CO_2}, as occurs during respiratory alkalosis (eg, high altitude hyperventilation), causes a decrease in secretion. The effects are not due to the CO_2 molecule itself but to the effects of an altered Pa_{CO_2} on renal intracellular pH. Thus, because the tubular membranes are quite permeable to CO_2, an increased arterial P_{CO_2} causes an equivalent increase in P_{CO_2} within the tubular cells. This, in turn, causes, by production of bicarbonate and hydrogen ion from water and CO_2, elevated intracellular hydrogen ion concentration, and it is this change that, via a sequence of intracellular events, increases the rate of hydrogen ion secretion. This probably occurs in most, if not all, the tubular segments that secrete hydrogen ions.

The second signal that influences hydrogen ion secretion in a homeostatic manner is a change in extracellular pH unrelated to Pa_{CO_2}. The generalization is that a decreased extracellular pH acts directly on the tubular cells, at least in part by changing intracellular pH, to stimulate hydrogen ion secretion. An increased extracellular pH does the opposite. As with Pa_{CO_2}, these effects are probably exerted on most, if not all, the tubular segments that secrete hydrogen ions.

We can see that these renal responses are appropriate. If the Pa_{CO_2} is high (causing a drop in plasma pH), the increased hydrogen ion secretion raises plasma bicarbonate, thereby restoring plasma pH to normal (despite the continued high Pa_{CO_2}). Similarly, if the pH is low because of low bicarbonate, the new bicarbonate restores the bicarbonate (and, therefore, the pH) to normal.

CONTROL OF RENAL GLUTAMINE METABOLISM AND NH$_4^+$ EXCRETION

In addition to regulating hydrogen ion secretion per se, there are several homeostatic controls over the production and tubular handling of NH_4^+. First, the generation of glutamine by the liver is increased by low extracellular pH. In this case, the liver shifts some of the disposal of ammonium ion from urea to glutamine. Second, the

---

[7] Here again, misuse of the "-osis" versus "-emia" suffixes can confuse the reader. A respiratory acidosis, as described later, simply means a high P_{CO_2} (> 40 mm Hg). It does *not* mean that CO_2 is entering the body at an elevated rate. If the P_{CO_2} is high but bicarbonate is normal, then, by the Henderson-Hasselbalch equation, the pH must be low.

Table 9–3. Homeostatic control of the processes that determine renal compensations for acid base disturbances

1	Glutamine metabolism and NH_4^+ excretion are increased during acidosis and decreased during alkalosis. The signal is unknown.
2	Tubular hydrogen ion secretion is
	a Increased by the increased blood P_{CO_2} of respiratory acidosis and decreased by the decreased P_{CO_2} of respiratory alkalosis.
	b Increased, independently of changes in P_{CO_2}, by the local effects of decreased extracellular pH on the tubules; the opposite is true for increased extracellular pH.

renal metabolism of glutamine is also subject to physiological control by extracellular pH. A decrease in extracellular pH stimulates renal glutamine oxidation by the proximal tubule, whereas an increase does just the opposite. Thus, an acidosis, by stimulating renal glutamine oxidation, causes the kidneys to contribute more new bicarbonate to the blood, thereby counteracting the acidosis. This pH responsiveness increases over the first few days of an acidosis and allows the glutamine–NH_4^+ mechanism for new bicarbonate generation to become the predominant renal process for opposing the acidosis. Conversely, an alkalosis inhibits glutamine metabolism, resulting in little or no renal contribution of new bicarbonate via this route.

In conclusion, acidosis increases renal NH_4^+ synthesis and excretion, whereas alkalosis does the opposite. This explains the spectrum of changes in NH_4^+ excretion summarized previously. These effects are summarized in Table 9–3.

INTRAVENOUS SOLUTIONS: LACTATED RINGER'S

One more way in which acid-base loads can enter the body is via intravenous solutions. Hospitalized patients receive a variety of intravenous solutions, the most common being physiological saline (0.9% NaCl) and 5% dextrose monohydrate (D_5W). Physiological saline is iso-osmotic with normal body fluids (osmolality, 287 mOsm/kg), whereas D_5W is slightly hypotonic (osmolality, 263 mOsm/kg). Neither has any acid-base content. Another common solution is lactated Ringer's solution, a mixture of salts that contains lactate at a concentration of 28 mEq/L. The pH is about 6.5. However, this is an *alkalinizing* solution for the same reason described as the fruit juice paradox earlier. Lactate is the conjugate base of lactic acid. When lactate is oxidized to CO_2 and water, it takes a hydrogen ion from the body fluids (and leaves a bicarbonate).[8]

Table 9–4 provides a summary of the processes, other than CO_2 production, of adding acids and bases to the body fluids. We omit CO_2 production because, except for transient states, CO_2 production is always matched by CO_2 excretion via the lungs. The unifying and, therefore, simplifying principle is that all processes of acid or base

---

[8] The effect of lactated Ringer's (alkalinizes the body) should not be confused with a lactic acidosis (acidifies the body) associated with exercise. A lactic acidosis results from the anaerobic conversion of glucose to lactic acid (lactate plus a hydrogen ion), whereas lactated Ringer's solution contains only lactate.

Table 9–4. Summary of processes that acidify or alkalinize the blood

Nonrenal mechanisms of acidifying the blood
  Consumption and metabolism of protein (meat) containing acidic or sulfur-containing amino
    acids
  Consumption of acidic drugs
  Metabolism of substrate without complete oxidation (fat to ketones and carbohydrate to lactic
    acid).
  GI tract secretion of bicarbonate (puts acid in blood)

Nonrenal machanisms of alkalinizing the blood
  Consumption and metabolism of fruit and vegetables containing basic amino acids or the salts of
    weak acids
  Consumption of antacids
  Infusion of lactated Ringer's solution
  GI tract secretion of acid (puts bicarbonate in the blood)

Renal mechanisms of acidifying the blood
  Allow some filtered bicarbonate to pass into the urine
  Secrete bicarbonate (Type B intercalated cells)

Renal means of alkalinizing the blood
  Secrete protons that form urine titratable acidity (Type A intercalated cells)
  Excrete NH_4^+ synthesized from glutamine

GI, gastrointestinal.

addition boil down to addition or loss of bicarbonate. All processes that acidify the blood end up removing bicarbonate, and all processes that alkalinize the blood end up adding bicarbonate.

SPECIFIC CATEGORIES OF ACID-BASE DISORDERS

To help sort out the many acid-base disorders, clinicians assign them to 4 categories: (1) respiratory acidosis, (2) respiratory alkalosis, (3) metabolic acidosis, and (4) metabolic alkalosis. For reference, we again write this in the form of the Henderson-Hasselbalch equation for the CO_2–bicarbonate buffer system.

$$pH = 6.1 + \log [\text{bicarbonate}]/ 0.03 \, P_{CO_2}$$

The definition of acid-base disorders is simple conceptually. If there are respiratory disorders, the Pa_{CO_2} is high or low; if there are metabolic disorders, the bicarbonate is high or low. As we see in the Henderson-Hasselbalch equation, changing the Pa_{CO_2} or changing the bicarbonate concentration raises or lowers the pH.

 In a respiratory acidosis (eg, resulting from pulmonary insufficiency), the low ventilation causes an increase in Pa_{CO_2}, in turn causing a decrease in pH.[9]

---

[9] The reader is reminded that this does not mean the body is being flooded with CO_2 that is somehow retained. Although there was a *transient* period of CO_2 accumulation to raise the P_{CO_2}, the patient with a respiratory P_{CO_2} disorder is not producing CO_2 faster than normal nor eliminating it slower than normal.

It should be clear from the Henderson-Hasselbalch equation that the pH could be restored to normal if the bicarbonate could be elevated to the same degree as the elevation in $Paco_2$. It is the kidneys' job to cause this bicarbonate increase by contributing new bicarbonate to the blood. An elevation in bicarbonate in response to an altered $Paco_2$ is called *compensation*. Compensation occurs because (1) NH_4^+ production and excretion are increased by the acidosis and (2) the increase in $Paco_2$ and drop in extracellular pH both stimulate renal tubular hydrogen ion secretion so that all filtered bicarbonate is reabsorbed, and increased amounts of secreted hydrogen ion are left over for the formation of titratable acid.

Renal compensation varies in effectiveness. If the elevation in bicarbonate is great enough to bring the pH back to within the normal range, the situation is well compensated. Generally, compensation is not complete (ie, when a new steady state is reached, the plasma bicarbonate is usually not elevated to quite the same degree as the $Paco_2$). Consequently, blood pH is not returned completely to normal. If the pH remains quite low, this is a uncompensated or partially compensated case. Note that with a well-compensated case, even though the pH does not indicate that something is wrong, the elevated $Paco_2$ and elevated bicarbonate indeed indicate that things are not normal.

The renal compensation in response to respiratory alkalosis is just the opposite. Respiratory alkalosis is the result of hyperventilation, in which the person *transiently* eliminates carbon dioxide faster than it is produced, thereby lowering $Paco_2$ and raising pH. Thereafter, even though ventilation remains high, CO_2 production and its excretion are normal. The decreased $Paco_2$ and increase in extracellular pH reduce tubular hydrogen ion secretion, so that bicarbonate reabsorption is not complete. In addition, bicarbonate secretion is stimulated. Bicarbonate is, therefore, lost from the body, and the loss results in decreased plasma bicarbonate and a return of plasma pH toward normal. There is no titratable acid in the urine (the urine is alkaline in these conditions), and there is little or no NH_4^+ in the urine because the alkalosis inhibits NH_4^+ production and excretion.

RENAL RESPONSE TO METABOLIC ACIDOSIS AND ALKALOSIS

A metabolic alkalosis or metabolic acidosis occurs when there is a high or low bicarbonate level. There are many possible causes of metabolic disturbances, including the kidneys themselves. The primary basis for the decrease in bicarbonate in metabolic acidosis is the addition to the body of increased amounts of any acid other than CO_2 (ie, a fixed acid) by ingestion, infusion, or production; decreased renal production of bicarbonate (as in renal failure); or direct loss of bicarbonate from the body (as in diarrhea). The result is the same regardless of whether there is loss of bicarbonate or addition of hydrogen ions: a lower concentration of bicarbonate and a lower plasma pH. The kidneys' response is an attempt to raise the plasma bicarbonate concentration back toward normal, thereby returning pH toward normal. To do this, the kidneys must reabsorb all the filtered bicarbonate and contribute new bicarbonate through increased formation and excretion of NH_4^+ and titratable acid. This is precisely what normal kidneys do, but if the acid load is too great or the problem is in the kidneys themselves, the bicarbonate concentration will remain low.

Just as there is renal compensation for a respiratory acid-base disturbance, there is *respiratory* compensation for a metabolic disturbance. Specifically, a decrease in arterial pH stimulates ventilation, thereby lowering $PaCO_2$, whereas a rise in arterial pH retards ventilation, allowing $PaCO_2$ to rise.

By now the astute reader has recognized a potential problem in the interpretation of acid-base disorders. When any acid-base disorder is well compensated, both the $PaCO_2$ and bicarbonate are elevated or depressed in the same direction (eg, in a well-compensated respiratory acidosis, both the $PaCO_2$ and bicarbonate are high). Thus, is this actually a respiratory acidosis with renal compensation, or is it a metabolic alkalosis with respiratory compensation? Similarly, in a well-compensated metabolic acidosis, both the $PaCO_2$ and bicarbonate are low. However, in a real-life situation, renal compensation for respiratory acid-base disturbances can be nearly complete, whereas respiratory compensation is usually only partial (after all, we cannot afford to stop breathing to correct blood pH). In addition, it would be rare in a clinical setting not to have additional information. For example, the high $PaCO_2$ of an emphysema patient is, in all likelihood, a respiratory acidosis resulting from impaired ventilation, not a compensation for a metabolic alkalosis. Nevertheless, real-life mixed acid-base disorders often present a challenge in the clinic.

FACTORS CAUSING THE KIDNEYS TO GENERATE OR MAINTAIN A METABOLIC ALKALOSIS

Rarely, otherwise normally functioning kidneys transport hydrogen ions *inappropriately* and thereby either generate or maintain an acid-base disorder, in this case metabolic alkalosis. In any metabolic alkalosis, the plasma bicarbonate concentration is elevated. This problem is not a defect in the ability of the kidneys to excrete bicarbonate; if a person is fed a large load of bicarbonate, the kidneys can excrete the load without a major rise in bicarbonate levels. The problem seems to be in *regulation* of bicarbonate excretion. The most important situations in which this occurs are (1) volume contraction, (2) chloride depletion, and (3) the combination of aldosterone excess and potassium depletion. The key event in all these situations is oversecretion of hydrogen ion (and sometimes of NH_4^+ as well), producing a metabolic alkalosis, or failing to respond as usual to an existing metabolic alkalosis.

Influence of Extracellular Volume Contraction

The presence of total-body volume contraction, because of salt loss, interferes with the ability of the kidneys to handle bicarbonate appropriately. Because the bicarbonate concentration is high in any metabolic alkalosis, the normal renal response should be to set hydrogen ion secretion at a level that falls short of complete bicarbonate reabsorption, thereby allowing the excess bicarbonate to be excreted. However, the presence of the extracellular volume contraction stimulates not only sodium reabsorption but also hydrogen ion secretion presumably because of high circulating levels of aldosterone. The generation or maintenance of a metabolic alkalosis in volume contraction may also occur when the volume is normal or high but the body "thinks" volume is low, specifically in congestive heart failure and advanced liver cirrhosis.

In volume contraction, the renin-angiotensin system is usually activated, resulting in stimulation of aldosterone secretion. Besides stimulating sodium reabsorption, aldosterone stimulates hydrogen ion secretion by Type A intercalated cells. The net result is that all the filtered bicarbonate is reabsorbed so that the already elevated plasma bicarbonate associated with the preexisting metabolic alkalosis is locked in, and the plasma pH remains high. The urine, instead of being alkaline, as it should be when the kidneys are normally responding to a metabolic alkalosis, is somewhat acid.

Influence of Chloride Depletion

We referred to extracellular volume contraction without distinguishing between sodium and chloride losses as the cause because loss of either of these ions will lead to extracellular volume contraction. However, we emphasize that specific chloride depletion, in a manner independent of and in addition to extracellular volume contraction, helps maintain metabolic alkalosis by stimulating hydrogen ion secretion. The most common reasons for chloride depletion are chronic vomiting and heavy use of diuretics. The result is that bicarbonate excretion remains essentially zero, and the metabolic alkalosis is not corrected.

Influence of Aldosterone Excess and Simultaneous Potassium Depletion

As noted, aldosterone stimulates hydrogen ion secretion. Potassium depletion, by itself, also weakly stimulates tubular hydrogen ion secretion and NH_4^+ production. However, the combination of potassium depletion of even moderate degree and high levels of aldosterone stimulates tubular hydrogen ion secretion markedly (NH_4^+ production also goes up significantly). As a result, the renal tubules not only reabsorb all filtered bicarbonate but also contribute inappropriately large amounts of new bicarbonate to the body, thereby causing metabolic alkalosis. Note that there may have been nothing wrong with the acid-base balance to start with: The alkalosis is actually generated by the kidneys themselves. Of course, if alkalosis were already present, this high aldosterone-potassium depletion combination would not only prevent the kidneys from responding appropriately but would also make the alkalosis worse. This phenomenon is important because the combination of a markedly elevated aldosterone and potassium depletion occurs in a variety of clinical situations, the most common of which is the extensive use of diuretic drugs (eg, from extensive, inappropriate diuretic use for weight loss) that can generate a metabolic alkalosis Figure 9–9.

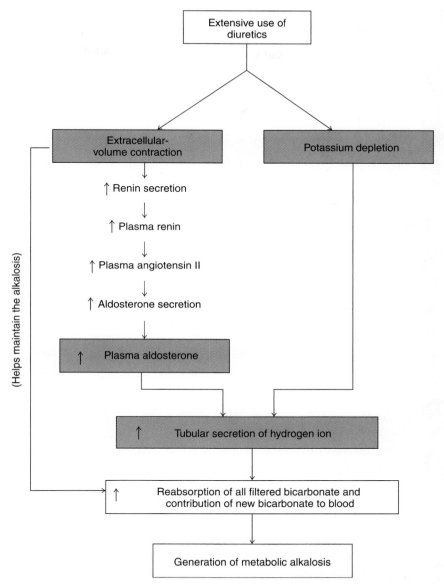

Figure 9–9. Pathway by which overuse of diuretics leads to a metabolic alkalosis. NH_4^+ production and excretion are also increased by the presence of a high aldosterone and potassium depletion. The extracellular volume contraction, via both aldosterone and as yet unidentified nonaldosterone mechanisms, helps to maintain the alkalosis once it has been generated. If the diuretics have also caused chloride depletion, this too will contribute to the maintenance of the metabolic alkalosis (not shown).

KEY CONCEPTS

 To maintain acid-base balance, the kidneys must excrete acid or base at a rate that matches net input.

 The regulation of body pH consists of regulating the concentrations of CO_2 (P_{CO_2}) and bicarbonate.

 The addition or loss of fixed acids and bases is equivalent to removing or adding bicarbonate.

 Fixed acids and bases can enter the body via GI processes, metabolism, intravenous infusions, and renal processes.

 Under all conditions, the kidneys must recover virtually all filtered bicarbonate proximally and then add acid or base distally depending on input.

 The kidneys excrete acid by titrating (acidifying) filtered base.

 The kidneys also excrete acid by converting glutamine to bicarbonate and ammonium, excreting the ammonium, and returning the bicarbonate to the blood.

 Primary acid-base disorders that change either P_{CO_2} or bicarbonate can be compensated by changing the other variable in the same direction, thereby preserving the ratio of bicarbonate to P_{CO_2}.

 Some situations, including volume contraction and aldosterone excess, can cause the kidneys to excrete too much acid, generating a metabolic alkalosis.

 ## STUDY QUESTIONS

9–1. Even if the urine pH is neutral (7.4), the kidneys can still excrete acid in the form of ammonium. True or false?

9–2. A patient is observed to excrete 2 L of alkaline (pH, 7.6) urine having a bicarbonate concentration of 28 mmol/L. What is the rate of titratable acid excretion?

    A. 56 mmol

    B. Negative

    C. Cannot determine without data for ammonium

9–3. Which of the following is an acid load per se or generates an acid load that must be excreted by the kidneys?

A. Prolonged vomiting of stomach secretions

B. Eating unsweetened grapefruit juice

C. Eating sweetened grapefruit juice

D. Intravenous infusion of sodium lactate

9–4. Proximal tubular reabsorption of filtered bicarbonate involves a pair of transporters: one that imports bicarbonate across the apical membrane and another that exports bicarbonate across the basolateral membrane. True or false?

9–5. During a metabolic acidosis, such as a diabetic ketoacidosis, the renal excretion of acid decreases well below normal levels. True or false?

9–6. Two patients have plasma pH values of 7.39 and 7.41, respectively. What is their acid-base status?

A. One is acidotic; the other is alkalotic.

B. They are both normal.

C. There is not enough information.

9–7. An emphysema patient has had serious difficulty breathing for a long time. Which of the situations below are likely?

A. His P_{CO_2} is elevated.

B. His bicarbonate is low.

C. His urine has an elevated amount of titratable acidity.

9–8. From an acid-base perspective, 1 mEq of titratable acid in the urine is the same as 1 mmol of ammonium. True or false?

Regulation of Calcium and Phosphate Balance

10

OBJECTIVES

The student understands body calcium balance and how the kidneys participate in regulation:

▶ *State the normal total plasma calcium concentration and the fraction that is free.*
▶ *Describe the distribution of calcium between bone and extracellular fluid and the role of bone in regulating extracellular calcium.*
▶ *Describe and compare the roles of the gastrointestinal tract and kidneys in calcium balance.*
▶ *Describe and compare osteocytic osteolysis and bone remodeling.*
▶ *Describe the role of vitamin D in calcium balance.*
▶ *Describe the synthesis of the active form of vitamin D (calcitriol) and how it is regulated.*
▶ *Describe the regulation of parathyroid hormone secretion and state the major actions of parathyroid hormone.*

The student understands body phosphate balance and how the kidneys participate in regulation:

▶ *Describe renal handling of phosphate.*
▶ *Describe how parathyroid hormone changes renal phosphate excretion.*

Calcium is a substance essential for a wide variety of body functions. Although calcium obeys the principles of input–output balance (as do all the other substance we have discussed), regulation of plasma calcium is fundamentally different from other substances we have considered because its balance is regulated by the gastrointestinal (GI) tract as well as the kidney. In addition, like potassium, plasma calcium is strongly "buffered" by large amounts of calcium (mostly in bone) that is readily exchangeable with extracellular fluid (ECF) calcium.

There are 2 time scales of calcium balance to consider: rapid transfer of calcium between the ECF and other tissues of the body and the slow rate of calcium ingestion into and excretion from the body. Calcium in the ECF represents only a tiny fraction of total-body calcium, but its level is crucial for the function of excitable cells in the body. Thus, it is essential to maintain the concentration of free calcium in our ECF within a narrow range. Too low a concentration leads to the life-threatening condition of low-calcium tetany (discussed later). Moment-to-moment regulation of extracellular calcium is achieved not by balancing input with renal excretion but rather by shifting calcium in and out of bone.

Bone stores of calcium serve as an enormous buffer system capable of taking up excess input and supplying calcium when there is no input.

In essence, balance for calcium in the ECF is balance to and from bone, not the outside world. Besides the rapid exchange of calcium into or out of bone, there is also a long-term regulation of total calcium in bone. Here the kidneys play an important but indirect role because they excrete some calcium in the urine and are involved in forming the active form of vitamin D. However, the dominant regulation of total-body calcium balance is less focused on output and more focused on input from the GI tract. Interestingly, and in contrast to most substances considered thus far, absorption of dietary calcium is only partial. In fact, most calcium that we eat simply passes through the GI tract to the feces. Calcium is both reabsorbed and secreted in the gut. Secretory rate is more or less constant, but the fraction absorbed is regulated to produce anywhere from small to moderate net absorption. Some net absorption is essential for the long-term maintenance of adequate bone calcium. Lack of calcium during childhood growth leads to a weak bone condition called rickets, and loss of calcium in an adult leads to osteomalacia or osteoporosis.[1]

Normal levels of plasma calcium are about 10 mg/dL (2.5 mmol/L or 5 mEq/L). This calcium exists in 3 general forms. First, almost half is in the free ionized (Ca^{2+}) form. This is the only form that is biologically active in target organs. Second, about 15% is complexed to anions with relatively low molecular weights, such as citrate and phosphate. Third, the remaining 40% is reversibly bound to plasma proteins. Calcium in the ECF is the source for calcium entering cells through calcium channels and is the calcium that triggers exocytosis of hormone and neurotransmitters and signals contraction in smooth and cardiac muscle cells.

A second role of extracellular calcium is to regulate the threshold for excitation in nerve and muscle cells. This role is completely separate from its role as a cation that enters through membrane channels. Calcium binds reversibly to surface membranes and influences the electric field sensed by all voltage-gated channels, specifically including sodium channels. Low levels of calcium fool the channels into sensing more depolarization than actually exists, leading to spontaneous firing of motor neurons. In turn, this firing triggers inappropriate muscle contraction, called *low-calcium tetany*. If severe enough, it leads to respiratory arrest because of spasms in the ventilatory muscles. [2]

---

[1] Rickets, osteomalacia, and osteoporosis are characterized by low calcium content in bone. Rickets and osteomalacia are commonly associated with a low *supply* of calcium, typically because of low vitamin D. Osteoporosis seems to represent improper *regulation,* so that the ongoing bone-forming and bone-dissolving processes are dominated by bone dissolution.

[2] Even though calcium in the extracellular medium is required to trigger the release of neurotransmitter from motor neurons (absence of calcium blocks this process completely), low calcium causes excessive muscle stimulation because hyperexcitability is manifested at calcium levels well above the extremely low levels needed to block exocytosis.

One of the most important influences on the degree of calcium binding to nerve membranes is the plasma pH. Serum albumin has many anionic sites that reversibly bind protons and calcium. These ions compete for occupancy of the binding sites. As pH rises, protons dissociate and calcium ions take their place, thereby lowering the concentration of free calcium ions. In turn, this tends to cause reduced binding of calcium to cell membranes. Thus, a patient with an acute alkalosis is more susceptible to tetany, whereas someone with acidosis will not manifest tetany at levels of total plasma calcium low enough to cause symptoms in normal people.

EFFECTOR SITES FOR CALCIUM BALANCE

GI Tract

As mentioned, and in contrast to sodium, chloride, and potassium, most ingested calcium is not normally absorbed from the intestine and simply leaves the body along with the feces. Accordingly, changes in the active transport system that moves calcium from intestinal lumen to blood can result in large increases or decreases in calcium absorption. Hormonal control of this absorptive process is the major means for homeostatically regulating total-body calcium balance.

Kidneys

The kidneys handle calcium by filtration and reabsorption. About 60% of the plasma calcium is filterable; the remainder is bound to plasma proteins. Most calcium reabsorption occurs in the proximal tubule (about 60% of the filtered load) and the remainder in the thick ascending limb of Henle's loop, distal convoluted tubule, and collecting-duct system. Overall, reabsorption is normally 97–99%.

Calcium reabsorption in the proximal tubule and thick ascending limb of Henle's loop is largely passive and paracellular, and the electrochemical forces driving it are dependent directly or indirectly on sodium reabsorption. In contrast, calcium reabsorption in the more distal segments is active and transcellular. In the distal tubule, calcium enters across the luminal surface via calcium-specific channels and exits across the basolateral membrane actively by a combination of Ca–adenosine triphosphatase (ATPase) and Na-Ca antiport activity (Figure 10–1). The distal tubule is where endocrine control of renal calcium handling is exerted.

The amount of calcium excreted in the urine is, on average, equal to the net addition of new calcium to the body via the GI tract; thus, the kidneys help maintain a stable balance of total-body calcium. However, the change in renal excretion in response to changes in dietary input is much less than the equivalent responses to dietary sodium, water, or potassium. For example, only about 5% of an increment in dietary calcium appears in the urine, whereas virtually all of an increased ingestion of water or sodium soon appears in the urine. The reason is that most of the dietary increment never gains entry to the blood because it fails to be absorbed from the GI tract. In contrast, when dietary intake of calcium is reduced to extremely low levels, there is a slow reduction of urinary calcium, but some continues to appear in the urine for weeks.

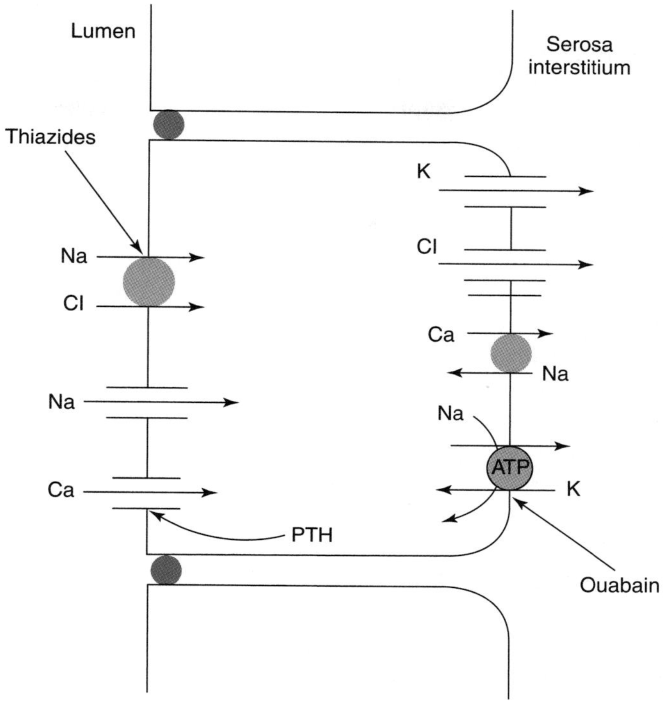

Figure 10–1. Major transport pathways in the distal convoluted tubule showing mechanisms of calcium reabsorption. The apical membrane contains the Na-Cl symporter (NCC), which is the target for inhibition by thiazide diuretics. Interestingly, inhibition of NCC with thiazide diuretics promotes calcium reabsorption (probably by enhancing the basolateral sodium gradient and increasing Na-Ca exchange). Thus, thazide may reduce the calcium loss associated with osteoporosis. There is also some sodium reabsorption via apical sodium channels (ENaCs). The DCT is also the major site for regulated reabsorption of Ca via apical Ca channels (under control of parathyroid hormone [PTH]) and a basolateral Na-Ca exchanger. A defect in NCC leads to Gitelman's syndrome, which, as might be expected, produces substantial diuresis, natriuresis, and kaliuresis but surprisingly is also characterized by hypocalciuria presumably because the activity of the Na-Ca antiporter is enhanced by low intracellular sodium, and the resultant low intracellular calcium acts as a driving force for apical reabsorption.

How do the renal homeostatic mechanisms operate? Because calcium is filtered and reabsorbed, but not secreted,

$$\text{Ca excretion} = \text{Ca filtered} - \text{Ca reabsorbed}$$

Accordingly, excretion can be altered homeostatically by changing either the filtered load or the rate of reabsorption. Both occur. For example, what happens when a person increases calcium intake? Transiently, intake exceeds output, positive calcium balance ensues, and plasma calcium concentration may increase. (However, recall that bone acts as a huge calcium buffer, so the rise in plasma calcium is slight.) A rise in plasma calcium increases both the filtered mass of calcium and excretion. Simultaneously, as we will see, the increased plasma calcium triggers hormonal changes that cause a diminished reabsorption. The net result of these responses is increased calcium excretion.

A wide variety of factors not designed to maintain calcium homeostasis can also influence urinary calcium excretion, mainly by stimulating or inhibiting tubular reabsorption. These include a large number of hormones, ions, acid-base disturbances, and drugs.

One of the most important of these influences on calcium reabsorption is sodium. An increase or decrease in urinary calcium excretion can be induced simply by administering or withholding salt, respectively. (This fact is used clinically when one wishes to decrease or increase the amount of calcium in the body.) The explanation is that, as described earlier, passive calcium reabsorption in the proximal tubule and thick ascending limb of Henle's loop is dependent on sodium reabsorption.

A second very important factor that influences tubular calcium reabsorption but is not designed to maintain calcium homeostasis is the presence of an acidosis. The mechanism is not clear, but acidosis markedly inhibits calcium reabsorption and, hence, causes increased calcium excretion. Alkalosis tends to do just the opposite: enhance calcium reabsorption and reduce excretion.

Bone

Bone is a complex tissue structurally and physiologically. It is the least understood, but in some ways the most important, of the major effector systems for calcium regulation. It is a major repository of calcium and serves as a crucial calcium-buffering system. About 0.5 g of calcium passes back and forth between bone and the blood plasma each day. The majority of the bone mass is made of a tough proteinaceous framework, mostly collagen, on which is deposited hard mineral crystals (hydroxyapatite). Hydroxyapatite is a complex of calcium, phosphate and hydroxyl ions.[3] Although very hard, bone is not uniformly solid like brick. Rather, it is penetrated by a labyrinth of tiny passageways containing fluid (bone fluid), cells (mostly osteocytes), and, in the larger passageways, blood vessels. The fluid in bone that is in direct contact with the hydroxyapatite is different in composition from blood plasma and ECF in other parts of the body. Surprisingly, it has a lower concentration of calcium (and a much higher concentration of potassium) than does plasma. All bone surfaces that are potential sites of communication between bone and the blood plasma are covered by a lining of cells (called "bone membrane") that separates bone fluid from other fluids in the body. These cells are mostly flattened versions of the active osteoblasts involved in forming bone. Details of the transport processes across the bone membrane are lacking, but the movement of calcium from bone fluid to plasma is up a concentration gradient and, therefore, must involve an active transport step.

---

[3] Apatites are a class of compounds of variable structural formula that usually include calcium, phosphate, and an anion such as fluoride, chloride, or hydroxide. The apatites in bone are a mixture of these, but the dominant one is hydroxyapatite

It is believed that the osteocytes deep within bone communicate with each other and the surface cells via long cellular extensions interfaced to each other by gap junctions. Calcium can be moved back and forth between blood and the inner recesses of bone via this cellular network.

Movement of calcium across the bone membrane constitutes the rapid buffering system that protects the blood plasma from major swings in calcium concentration. This process is often called *osteocytic osteolysis.* There is a second flux process involving calcium, called bone *remodeling,* that affects bone structure in the long term but is not directly involved in rapidly regulating plasma calcium. Remodeling involves giant, multinucleated cells called *osteoclasts* that erode little pits in the bone matrix. Nearby, osteoblasts follow behind and fill in the pits with new bone matrix. The daily flux of calcium via remodeling is less than that associated with osteocytic osteolysis across the bone membrane, but imbalance in the remodeling process over a long period of time generates bone pathology such as osteoporosis.

HORMONAL CONTROL OF EFFECTOR SITES

The regulation of calcium is achieved mostly through the actions of 2 hormones: the active form of vitamin D—$1,25\text{-}(OH)_2D$—and parathyroid hormone (PTH), a peptide hormone produced by the parathyroid glands. The active form of vitamin D acts mainly to stimulate intestinal absorption of calcium and phosphate. In growing children, this ensures a supply of substrate for bone formation, and in adults it ensures a supply to replace the ongoing dissolution of bone. PTH has several actions, a key one being to dissolve bone and move calcium into the blood. PTH stimulates the bone membrane to move calcium on a short-term basis, and via paracellular signals from osteoblasts, also stimulates osteoclasts to resorb bone (Figure 10–2). These processes protect the body from low-calcium tetany. Simply stated, the active form of vitamin D regulates what comes into the body and PTH regulates what is in the ECF.

Vitamin D

The term vitamin D denotes a family of closely related molecules that are derived from cholesterol. One member of this family, called vitamin D_3 (cholecalciferol), is synthesized by the action of ultraviolet radiation on 7-dehydrocholesterol in the skin. The 7-dehydrocholesterol precursor is normally present in adequate amounts to avoid limiting the production of vitamin D_3. Thus, the synthesis of vitamin D_3 itself is strongly dependent on exposure to sunlight, which is, in turn, dependent on climate, latitude, clothing, and so on. Vitamin D_3, like cholesterol, is a 27-carbon molecule containing 1 hydroxyl group. Another member of the family is vitamin D_2, which is ingested in food, specifically food derived from plants. Vitamin D_2 (ergocalciferol) differs chemically from vitamin D_3 by an additional methyl group and a double bond between 2 of the carbons. It is the form of vitamin D usually added as a supplement to foods. These 2 members of the vitamin D family act identically. Vitamin D means either vitamin D_2 or vitamin D_3.

Vitamin D as such is inactive (ie, neither ingested vitamin D_2 nor the vitamin D_3 formed in the skin has any significant biological activity). It must undergo metabolic

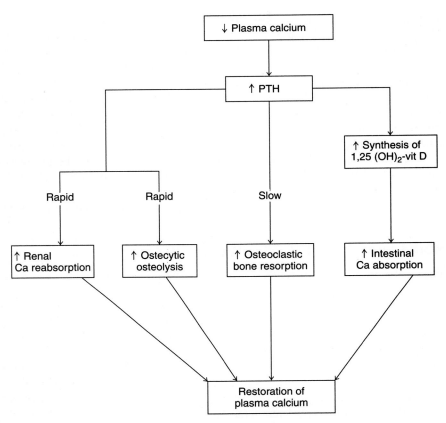

Figure 10–2. Response to reduced plasma calcium concentration. Parathyroid hormone (PTH) secretion increases acutely in response to a drop in plasma calcium concentration. PTH stimulates osteocytic osteolysis immediately, followed by increased renal calcium reabsorption. On a slower time scale, osteoclastic bone resorption increases, and increased synthesis of calcitriol in the kidney leads to increased absorption of dietary calcium from the GI tract.

changes within the body before it can influence its target cells. Circulating vitamin D is hydroxylated at the 25 position by the liver and then hydroxylated again at the 1 position by proximal tubular cells within the kidneys to yield a cholesterol derivative containing 3 hydroxyl groups. (When formed from vitamin D_3, it is called *calcitriol*. This is the form of vitamin D—1,25-dihydroxyvitamin D, or 1,25-$(OH)_2D$—that exerts actions on target cells. From this description, it should be evident that the molecular species that is actually exerting actions on target tissues is a hormone, not a vitamin, because it is made in the body. Therefore, we usually call this hormone the *active* form of vitamin D.

The major action of calcitriol is to stimulate active absorption of calcium and phosphate by the intestine. Details of how calcium is absorbed and how calcitriol regulates it are unclear. However, calcium probably enters from the intestinal lumen passively through calcium-selective channels, binds reversibly to mobile cytosolic calcium-binding proteins (called *calbindins*) that allow calcium to move across the cell without raising the concentration of free calcium, and then is actively transported out the basolateral side via a Ca-ATPase. A role of calcitriol is to stimulate synthesis of the proteins involved in these steps. In addition, calcitriol has some independent actions on bone that are not entirely clear. As well, calcitriol stimulates the renal-tubular reabsorption of calcium and phosphate. The influences of calcitriol on bone and the kidney are far less important than its actions on the GI tract to stimulate absorption of calcium and phosphate.

The major event in vitamin D deficiency is decreased gut calcium absorption, resulting in decreased availability of calcium for bone formation or reformation. In children, the newly formed bone protein matrix fails to be calcified normally because of the low availability of calcium, leading to the disease rickets.

PTH

The GI tract, kidneys, and bone are subject to direct or indirect control by PTH. Its half-life in the plasma is very short (< 10 min), and its secretion is controlled on a moment-to-moment basis by the calcium concentration of the ECF bathing the cells of the parathyroid glands. Decreased plasma calcium concentration stimulates PTH secretion, and increased plasma concentration inhibits secretion. Extracellular calcium concentration acts directly on the parathyroid glands by binding to a novel class of G protein–linked receptors whose ligands are divalent cations. The calcium receptor couples via an intracellular G protein to a signaling cascade that inhibits the secretion of PTH. Thus, low extracellular calcium stimulates PTH secretion by removing a tonic inhibition. This is a sensitive control system designed to keep free plasma calcium at about 5 mg/dL.

Phosphate also affects PTH secretion: Elevated phosphate stimulates PTH secretion by stimulating the capacity of the parathyroid gland to synthesize PTH, so that chronically high levels of phosphate lead to elevated PTH. Calcitriol has slower inhibitory effects (discussed later), but calcium is the primary *acute* regulator.

PTH exerts at least 4 distinct effects on calcium homeostasis (summarized in Figure 10–2):

1. It increases the movement of calcium from bone into ECF by stimulating bone osteocytic osteolysis (the rapid calcium retrieval process) and the slow resorption carried out by osteoclasts. In this manner, the immense store of calcium contained in bone is made available for the regulation of extracellular calcium concentration.

2. PTH stimulates the activation of vitamin D as described earlier (and this hormone then increases intestinal absorption of calcium). The blood concentration of calcitriol is subject to physiological control by PTH. The major control point is the second hydroxylation step, the one that occurs in the kidneys. This step

is stimulated by PTH. This action is highly adaptive. If plasma calcium falls, the subsequent increase in PTH immediately stimulates calcium transport from bone, thus restoring plasma calcium levels, and also stimulates calcium uptake (via calcitriol) from the GI tract. This ensures that enough new calcium will enter the body to replace that "borrowed" from bone.

3.   PTH increases renal-tubular calcium reabsorption, mainly by an action on the distal convoluted tubule. At this location, it increases apical membrane calcium entry through calcium channels. The increased uptake of calcium from the lumen stimulates basolateral extrusion (by a combination of Ca-ATPase activity and Na-Ca antiporter activity) and thus decreases urinary calcium excretion.[4]

4.   It *reduces* the proximal tubular reabsorption of phosphate, thereby raising urinary phosphate excretion and lowering extracellular phosphate concentration.

The adaptive value of the first 3 effects should be obvious: They all result in a higher extracellular calcium concentration and thus compensate for the lower calcium concentration that originally stimulated PTH secretion. Regarding the fourth effect, when PTH acts on bone, both calcium and phosphate are released into the blood.

Similarly, the active form of vitamin D enhances the intestinal absorption of both calcium and phosphate. Accordingly, the processes that are restoring calcium to its normal level are simultaneously tending to raise the plasma phosphate above normal. However, plasma phosphate does not actually increase because of PTH's *inhibition* of tubular phosphate reabsorption. Indeed, this effect is so potent that plasma phosphate may actually decrease when PTH levels are elevated. The simultaneous presence of high levels of both calcium and phosphate can create pathologies in a number of tissues, including the heart and blood vessels, because this increases the formation of insoluble calcium phosphate complexes.[5]

In contrast to the state described previously, an increase in extracellular calcium concentration reduces PTH secretion, thereby producing increased urinary and fecal calcium loss and net movement of calcium from ECF into bone.

PTH has other functions in the body, but the 4 effects discussed previously constitute the major mechanisms by which it integrates various organs and tissues in the regulation of extracellular calcium concentration.

Primary hyperparathyroidism, resulting from a primary defect in the parathyroid glands (eg, a hormone-secreting tumor), illustrates the actions of PTH. The excess

---

[4] The strongest and most commonly prescribed diuretics (called "loop" diuretics because they inhibit sodium reabsorption in the thick ascending limb of the loop of Henle) have the secondary effect of also decreasing calcium absorption. Another class of diuretics, called the thiazides, are somewhat weaker diuretics. They inhibit sodium reabsorption not in the loop but in the distal tubule by blocking the Na-Cl symporter. Interestingly, they *increase* Ca reabsorption by a mechanism that hyperpolarizes the cells and stimulates influx of Ca across the apical membrane.

[5] The chemistry of the Ca phosphates is complex because Ca and phosphate can combine in different stochiometric ratios, and the tendency of any of these to precipitate depends on the concentrations not only of Ca and phosphate but of other substances as well.

hormone causes enhanced bone resorption, leading to bone thinning and the formation of completely calcium-free areas or cysts. Plasma calcium increases and plasma phosphate decreases; the latter is caused by increased urinary phosphate excretion. The increased plasma calcium is deposited in various body tissues, including the kidneys, where stones may be formed. A seeming paradox is that urinary calcium excretion is *increased* despite the fact that tubular calcium reabsorption is enhanced by PTH. The reason is that the elevated plasma calcium concentration induced by the effects of PTH on bone (and via calcitriol on the load of calcium entering the body from the GI tract) causes the filtered load of calcium to increase even more than the reabsorptive rate. Because the filtered load is so great, there is also an increased amount *not* reabsorbed, (ie, excreted). This result nicely illustrates the necessity of taking both filtration and reabsorption (and secretion, if relevant) into account when analyzing excretory changes of any substance.

OVERVIEW OF RENAL PHOSPHATE HANDLING

The renal handling of phosphate has been mentioned almost always in the context of other topics, such as sodium reabsorption or urine acidification. We now review certain key aspects of renal phosphate handling because control of urinary phosphate excretion is a major pathway for the homeostatic regulation of total-body phosphate balance.

Approximately 5–10% of plasma phosphate is protein bound, so that 90–95% is filterable at the renal corpuscle. Normally, approximately 75% of this filtered phosphate is actively reabsorbed, almost entirely in the proximal tubule (in symport with sodium).

As with other substances handled by filtration and tubular reabsorption, the rate of phosphate excretion can be changed by altering the mass filtered per unit time or the mass reabsorbed per unit time. Indeed, even relatively small increases in plasma phosphate concentration (and, hence, filtered load) can produce relatively large increases in phosphate excretion. This occurs when plasma phosphate concentration increases as a result of increased dietary phosphate intake or release of phosphate from bone. Phosphate is reabsorbed by a tubular maximum-limited (T_m) system, and the normal filtered load is just a little higher than the T_m. Thus, most filtered phosphate is reabsorbed, but some spills into the urine. (Recall that this phosphate is responsible for accepting hydrogen ion in the collecting duct and is the primary ion responsible for titratable acidity.) This also means that the reabsorptive capacity is saturated at normal filtered loads, so any increase in filtered load simply adds to the amount excreted. As mentioned, systemic acidosis promotes release of calcium and phosphate from bone. The increase in plasma phosphate and consequently the filtered load of phosphate means that there is more titratable buffer in the collecting tubule to help remove the excess hydrogen ion that promoted the phosphate release.

Changes in PTH and calcitriol are not "designed" to mediate the homeostatic association between dietary phosphate and tubular phosphate reabsorption. Nevertheless, as we have seen, whenever parathyroid hormone is increased or decreased, tubular phosphate reabsorption is powerfully inhibited or stimulated, respectively. Other hormones, too, are known to alter phosphate reabsorption (eg, inulin increases it and glucagon decreases it).

Much of the physiology we have described is illustrated by the case of chronic renal failure, in which a low glomerular filtration rate limits the ability of the kidneys to excrete a number of substances, specifically phosphate. An almost universal complication of chronic renal failure is elevated plasma phosphate (hyperphosphatemia). Another common finding is elevated levels of PTH. The high PTH stimulates excessive bone resorption, leading to osteoporosis. This is an example of *secondary* hyperparathyroidism (not primary) because the pathology is not in the gland itself, but in the signals that drive it. One goal in the treatment of hyperphosphatemia associated with chronic renal failure is the reduction of phosphate absorption from the GI tract. This is accomplished by feeding the patient high doses of calcium. The calcium forms complexes with phosphate in the GI tract, reducing the availability of absorbable phosphate. The high levels of PTH in a normal patient *should* signal the kidneys to form calcitriol, but in chronic renal failure a further complication is a reduced ability to synthesize it. Another clinical intervention in this case is to provide exogenous calcitriol. This hormone suppresses expression of the PTH gene in the parathyroid gland. The calcitriol should increase GI absorption of phosphate, the very thing we are trying to inhibit, but its ability to lower the synthesis of PTH is more important because this reduces the excessive resorption of bone stimulated by PTH. Thus, administering calcitriol is a useful clinical tool.

KEY CONCEPTS

1. Moment-to-moment regulation of plasma calcium primarily involves calcium flux between bone and plasma rather than input and output from the body.

2. The most important action of vitamin D is to ensure adequate absorption of calcium from the GI tract.

3. PTH is essential both to maintain proper calcium flux between bone and plasma and to maintain adequate levels of vitamin D.

4. Keeping phosphate levels in the normal range allows normal calcium retrieval from bone.

STUDY QUESTIONS

10–1. The most important action of vitamin D is to stimulate:
  A. Calcium deposition in bone
  B. Calcium resorption from bone
  C. Calcium absorption from the GI tract
  D. Calcium reabsorption in the renal tubule

10–2. PTH stimulates phosphate secretion in the proximal tubule. True or false?

10–3. In response to a sudden decrease in plasma calcium, where does most of the calcium come from to restore plasma levels?
  A. The renal tubules
  B. Bone
  C. The GI tract

10–4. When calcium is resorbed from bone on a rapid basis, how does it get from bone crystal to blood plasma? Explain your answer.
  A. It simply diffuses out.
  B. It is taken up by osteoclasts.
  C. It is taken up by osteocytes.

Answers to Study Questions

CHAPTER 1

1–1. The correct answer is false. All glomeruli are in the cortex.

1–2. The correct answer is none. Most medullary blood is supplied by efferent arterioles near the corticomedullary border. A small fraction may be supplied from cortical radial arteries. All of these vessels are in the cortex.

1–3. The correct answer is no. It is possible that substance T was filtered, but substance T might also enter tubules by secretion into the tubules.

1–4. The correct answer is no. It is possible that it was neither secreted or filtered, but there is another possibility: Substance V may be filtered or secreted, but all the substance V entering the lumen via these routes may be completely reabsorbed. Many substances fall into this category.

1–5. The answer is none. In glomerular filtration, the filtered substances pass *around* the endothelial cells (through fenestrations) and around the podocytes. Topologically, Bowman's space is continuous with the external environment; thus, a filtered substance can move from blood to the bladder and be excreted without crossing through any plasma membrane.

1–6. The answer is no. *Freely filtered* means the substance is filtered in the same proportion that volume is filtered. If 20% of the volume is filtered, then 20% of a freely filtered substance is filtered, meaning that 80% is *not* filtered and passes on to the efferent arterioles and peritubular capillaries.

1–7. The answer is cortex. Cells of the macula densa are part of the juxtaglomerular apparatus, just next to the glomeruli that are all in the cortex.

1–8. The answer is yes. Under all circumstances, there is net volume reabsorption in the medulla. By mass balance, this requires that the reabsorbed volume leave the medulla. The only way out for reabsorbed substances is in the blood. Blood flow out is slightly greater than blood flow in.

CHAPTER 2

2–1. The answer is false. Freely filtered means no restriction or sieving by the filtration barrier. Because normally about 20% of the plasma volume is filtered, then about 20% of substance X would be filtered.

2–2. The answer is 125 mg/min. The amount of any substance filtered per unit time is given by the product of the GFR and the filterable plasma concentration of the substance, in this case, 125 mL/min × 100 mg/100 mL (1 dL = 100 mL).

2–3. Approximately 40% of the calcium in plasma is bound to proteins and so is not filterable.

2–4. If the protein were freely filtered, there would be 100 mg/L × 100 L/day = 10 g/day. However, no exact value can be calculated from these data because the molecular weight is high enough so that some "sieving" would occur. Some would be filtered, but not 10 g/day.

2–5. (1) Constrict glomerular mesangial cells and, hence, reduce K_f. (2) Lower arterial pressure and, hence, P_{GC}. (3) Constrict the afferent arteriole and, hence, reduce P_{GC}. (4) Dilate the efferent arteriole and, hence, reduce P_{GC}.

2–6. It might be increasing K_f (ie, changing the hydraulic permeability of the glomerular membranes or the surface area available for filtration).

2–7. RBF will show no change because the drug has no effect on total renal vascular resistance. GFR will increase because of a large increase in P_{GC}. Filtration fraction will, therefore, increase. (Now back up and think a bit more about the GFR: Because filtration fraction increases, there will be a larger than average increase in π_{GC} along the glomeruli, and this will offset some of the GFR-increasing effect of the increased P_{GC}, therefore, GFR will not increase as much proportionately as the P_{GC}.)

2–8. The answer is C. Arterial pressure decreases by 33%, but autoregulation prevents the RBF from decreasing in direct proportion. Autoregulation is not perfect, so some decrease, but not 33%, will occur.

CHAPTER 3

3–1. The answer is C. Clearance *units* are volume per time, not mass per time.

3–2. The answer is lower. Metabolic clearance rate includes all routes of elimination; its value is the renal clearance plus any others.

3–3. The answer is C. $C_{In} = U_{In}V/P_{In}$. When P_{In} increases, there is no change in C_{In} because U_{In} rises by an identical amount. In other words, the mass of inulin filtered and excreted increases, but the volume of plasma supplying this inulin (ie, completely cleared of inulin) is unaltered.

3–4. 1. Substance *A* is a large molecule poorly filtered at the glomerulus. 2. Substance *A* is bound, at least in part, to plasma protein. 3. Substance *A* is reabsorbed.

3–5. Substance *B* is secreted by the tubules.

3–6. PAH; creatinine; inulin; urea; sodium; glucose

3–7. The answer is 0.01. The excreted amount of sodium is as follows: 75 mmol/L × 2 mL/min × 0.001 L/ml = 0.15 mmol/min. Because sodium is freely filtered, the filtered amount is the GFR × P_{Na}, and GFR is the same as C_{In}. GFR = C_{In} = 50 mg/L ÷ 1 mg/L × 2 mL/min = 100 ml/min, or 0.1 L/min. Filtered sodium = 150 mmol/L × 0.1 L/min = 15 mmol/min. Therefore, the fraction of the filtered load that is excreted, fractional excretion, is 0.15 mmol/min ÷ 15 mmol/min = 0.01.

3–8. The answer is A.

CHAPTER 4

4–1.   The answer is false. Flux by a uniporter is always passive, down the electrochemical gradient. Flux by a symporter may be active depending on direction. Flux via an ATPase is always active. (Theoretically, it could pump downhill, but this does not normally occur.)

4–2.   Most regions of the nephron have tight junctions that are far less leaky than those found in the proximal tubule, and most apical membranes are far less permeable to water. As a result, it is possible to sustain much larger osmotic gradients across the epithelium in tubular regions beyond the proximal tubule. Reabsorption beyond the proximal tubule is generally not iso-osmotic.

4–3.   The answer is true.

4–4.   Failure to move fluid from the interstitium to peritubular capillary as a result of low plasma oncotic pressure quickly leads to an increased interstitial hydrostatic pressure because, at first, reabsorption proceeds normally. The interstitial space contains a small fraction of total volume of the kidneys, and only a small increase in fluid volume is required to generate a rise in hydrostatic pressure. Once interstitial pressure rises significantly, this drives an increasing back-leak.

4–5.   The answer is false. Not all solutes are alike osmotically. Proteins, for example, exert far more osmotic effect mole for mole than do saccharides. In addition, saccharides exert a somewhat higher osmotic effect than simple salts. In this text, we sometimes simplify things by using osmolarity, when technically we should use osmolality. In most cases, this does not introduce a large error.

4–6.   Despite the volume flow, most solutes are close to diffusional equilibrium between plasma and interstitium. If the interstitium starts to become depleted of a substance as a result of secretion, net diffusion from the plasma will soon replenish it.

4–7.   The answer is B. Normally, all the filtered glucose is reabsorbed, meaning that the filtered load does not saturate the transporters. If either A or C were true, there would be at least some glucose in the urine.

CHAPTER 5

5–1.   The answers are A, B, and C. These waste products are all normally excreted in large amounts; a decreased GFR would cause their plasma concentrations to increase until the filtered load was increased enough to reestablish normal excretion. In contrast, the reabsorption T_ms for glucose, amino acids, and many other organic compounds that are not waste products are usually so high relative to normal filtered loads that, even with a 50% loss of nephrons, virtually all the filtered loads are reabsorbed. Accordingly, their plasma concentrations are virtually independent of renal function (ie, the kidneys do not participate in the setting of their plasma concentrations).

5–2.   The answer is no. The overall tubular handling of urea is reabsorption. Urinary urea concentration is higher than that of plasma because relatively more water has been reabsorbed than urea, thereby concentrating the urea in the tubular fluid leaving the kidney.

5–3.   This is simply the GFR (180 L/day) times the concentration in the filtrate: 180 L/day × 0.005 g/dL × 10 dL/L = 9 g/day.

5–4.   The answer is A. The luminal membranes of nephron segments beyond the proximal tubule do not express glucose transporters, so no further reabsorption occurs regardless of conditions.

5–5.   Decreased pH (acidify the urine). This would convert more of the quinine to its charged form and prevent its passive reabsorption.

CHAPTER 6

6–1.   11.6 g/day.

6–2.   The answer is B. Mannitol is freely filtered and neither secreted nor reabsorbed. It acts as an excess osmole in the same way that glucose does when its filtered load exceeds the T_m for reabsorption. Sodium excretion will increase and for the same reasons as when there is excess glucose.

6–3.   The answer is true.

6–4.   The answer is true. Allowing back leak or chloride would reduce the paracellular reabsorption of sodium, and thus reduce the overall reabsorption of both sodium and chloride and prevent concentrating the medullary interstitium.

6–5.   The answer is false. There is no reabsorption of sodium or chloride by the descending thin limb of Henle's loop.

6–6.   The answer is true. There is always net reabsorption of both sodium and water in the medulla. Under the influence of ADH, there is further reabsorption of water in the inner medullary collecting ducts. This solute and water must be removed from the medullary interstitium.

6–7.   The answer is true. As with maximum levels of ADH, there is always net reabsorption of sodium and water in the medulla. With minimum levels of ADH, there is still net reabsorption of water in the inner medullary (not cortical) collecting ducts. As described in the text, with low levels of ADH (and hence little reabsorption in the cortex), the gradient for water reabsorption in the inner medulla is quite large, and there is always a finite water permeability in this region.

6–8.   It ceases completely. Even though the active step is not altered by the drug, there will be no sodium entering the cell to be acted on by the pumps.

CHAPTER 7

7–1.   (1) 5 mmol/min. Approximately two thirds of filtered sodium is reabsorbed by the proximal tubule. (2) 6.6 mmol/min. Filtered sodium rises from 15–20 mmol/min. Glomerulotubular balance maintains fractional sodium reabsorption at approximately two thirds of the filtered load.

7–2.   The answer is no. As soon as the person starts to become sodium deficient as a result of the increased sodium excretion, the usual sodium-retaining reflexes will be set into motion. They will, of course, be unable to raise aldosterone secretion, but they will lower GFR and alter the other factors that influence tubular sodium reabsorption to compensate at least partially for the decreased aldosterone-dependent sodium reabsorption.

7–3.   The answer is no. It will probably be above normal because of increased filtration fraction (ie, reduction in GFR and an even greater reduction in renal blood flow secondary to renal arteriolar constriction mediated by the renal sympathetic nerve and angiotensin II).

7–4.   The right kidney will have increased secretion because of decreased renal perfusion pressure acting via the intrarenal baroreceptor and decreased flow to the macula densa. This increased secretion will result in elevated systemic arterial angiotensin II and elevated arterial blood pressure, both of which will inhibit renin secretion from the left kidney.

7–5.   Plasma renin concentration is lower. The increased aldosterone causes the body to retain sodium, which reflexively inhibits renin secretion. Thus, one observes high plasma aldosterone and low plasma renin, a strong tip-off to the presence of the disease because, in almost all other situations, renin and aldosterone change in the same direction (because the renin-angiotensin system is the major control of aldosterone secretion).

7–6.   The answer is true. Although some diuretic drugs are more potent than others, blockage at any site results in at least mild diuresis. Because less than 2% of the filtered load is normally excreted, it does not require a huge reduction in the percentage reabsorbed to result in a large increase in the amount of sodium that is excreted.

7–7.   It will decrease. This question focuses on the effect of peritubular factors on proximal sodium reabsorption. The GFR will remain about the same, but the filtration fraction will decrease (total renal vascular resistance decreases, so renal blood flow increases). The peritubular capillary pressure will, therefore, rise. At the same time, the peritubular oncotic pressure will decrease because of the decreased filtration fraction. Both of these effects tend to reduce fluid reabsorption from the interstitium, which reduces proximal sodium and water reabsorption.

7–8.   There will be excess sodium. We cannot be sure of the net effect on water because there are opposing influences: the excess sodium leading to increased water excretion and the ADH-like effect leading to decreased water excretion. The osmolality, for sure, will be hyperosmotic.

7–9.   There will be excess sodium, excess water, and an iso-osmotic urine. Blocking sodium reabsorption in the thick ascending limb is what "loop diuretics" do. Not only do they lead to excess sodium and water in the urine, but they prevent the kidneys from generating a medullary osmotic gradient. Even with the ADH-like actions of the drug, the urine cannot become more concentrated than the now iso-osmotic medullary interstitium.

CHAPTER 8

8–1.   The answer is C: potassium secretion.

8–2.   For potassium, yes. High rates of secretion may exceed reabsorption. For sodium, no.

8–3.   A. False: Most potassium reabsorption is paracellular, but all sodium reabsorption is transcellular. B. True. C. False: Even though the multiporter moves equal amounts of sodium and potassium, most of the potassium leaks back and is recycled.

8–4.   The answer is true. The excess solute retains water, thus diluting tubular potassium and reducing the driving force for reabsorption.

8–5.   The answer is false. The high amounts of non-reabsorbed solute increase the sodium content of the luminal fluid, with water accompanying it. This dilutes potassium. This stimulates potassium secretion both by the dilution effect and by the high rate of sodium reabsorption.

8–6.   The answer is high. The increased aldosterone stimulates potassium secretion and, thereby, excretion. Moreover, once enough sodium has been retained to increase GFR and to cause partial inhibition of proximal reabsorption, the increased delivery of fluid to the cortical collecting duct further enhances potassium secretion. There is no potassium escape similar to the sodium escape from aldosterone.

8–7.   The answer is relatively normal. One may have answered "high," assuming that the increased aldosterone would stimulate potassium secretion, as in Question 8–6. However, this effect is more than balanced by the fact that the patient has a decrease in flow of fluid into the cortical collecting duct (because of decreased GFR and increased proximal and loop reabsorption). Recall that potassium secretion is impaired when the amount of fluid flowing through the cortical collecting duct is reduced. This explains why patients with the diseases of secondary hyperaldosteronism with edema do not lose large quantities of potassium, whereas those with primary hyperaldosteronism do.

CHAPTER 9

9–1.   The answer is true.

9–2.   The answer is B. If the urine has a pH greater than 7.4, clearly there is no titratable acid excreted. Indeed, there is negative titratable acid excretion. Ammonium does not contribute to titratable acid and may be ignored in the calculation of titratable acid.

9–3.   None of them are acid loads. Vomiting of stomach acid adds bicarbonate to the blood. Fruit juice, when oxidized to CO_2 and water, adds bicarbonate. Sweetening it makes no difference because the metabolism of saccharides is acid-base neutral. Lactate, when metabolized, adds bicarbonate.

9–4.   The answer is false. Filtered bicarbonate is not transported into the epithelial cells; rather, it is converted in the lumen to CO_2 and water when it combines with secreted protons. Bicarbonate is generated within the epithelium on a one-for-one basis as the secreted protons, and this bicarbonate is transported across the basolateral membrane.

9–5.   The answer is false. Renal acid excretion rises. The acidosis is caused by increased generation of metabolic acids, not failure of the kidneys to excrete acid. The kidneys respond by increasing their excretion of acid. A steady state is reached when input and output are both elevated and plasma bicarbonate is low.

9–6.   The answer is C. The pH values are both within the normal range, so both patients could be perfectly normal. However, pH is set by the *ratio* of bicarbonate to P_{CO_2}. Both values could be elevated or depressed, yielding a normal ratio but an acidosis or alkalosis that is well compensated.

9–7.   Answer A is certainly true. This a respiratory acidosis. Answer B is false. In response to the prolonged acidosis, the patient's bicarbonate would be elevated as compensation, not depressed. Answer C is false. Although the development of compensation would require increased acid excretion, the maintenance would only require a urinary excretion to match the input of fixed acid. CO_2, no matter how much it is elevated, cannot be excreted as urinary acid.

9–8.   The answer is true. The excretion of titratable acid and ammonium both involve secreting a hydrogen ion and generating a bicarbonate that goes into the blood.

CHAPTER 10

10–1.   The answer is C. Vitamin D probably acts in a permissive manner for all of these processes, but stimulation of calcium absorption from the GI tract is the most important direct action.

10–2.   The answer is false. PTH inhibits phosphate reabsorption, resulting in increased excretion. The increased excretion is the same result that *would* occur if secretion were increased, but phosphate is not secreted.

10–3.   The answer is B: bone.

10–4.   The answer is C. Rapid movement of calcium from bone to plasma is via osteocytic osteolysis. Calcium in bone is separated from calcium in plasma by "bone membrane," a cell layer of osteocytes and osteoblasts that prevents free diffusion but that transports calcium in both directions. Osteoclasts participate in bone remodeling, which is much slower than the rapid response to sudden changes in plasma calcium.

Appendix A

Table A-1. Summary of reabsorption and secretion by major tubular segments

	Proximal tubule		Henle's loop		Distal convoluted tubule		Collecting-duct system	
	R	S	R	S	R	S	R	S
Organic nutrients	X							
Urea	X			(X)			X	
Proteins, peptides	X							
Phosphate	X							
Sulfate	X							
Organic anions	X (can also be reabsorbed and/or secreted passively along tubule)							
Organic cations	X (can also be reabsorbed and/or secreted passively along tubule)							
Urate	X	X						
Sodium	X		X		X		X	
Chloride	X		X		X		X	
Water	X		X				X	
Potassium	X		X	(X)		X	X	X
Hydrogen ions		X		X		X		X
Bicarbonate	X		X		X		X	X
Ammonium	X	(X)						(X)
Calcium	X		X		X		X	

R, reabsorption; S, secretion.

Table A–2. Major functions of the various collecting-duct cells*

Principal cells

  1 Reabsorb sodium (stimulated by aldosterone).

  2 Secrete potassium (stimulated by aldosterone).

  3 Reabsorb water (stimulated by antidiuretic hormone).

Comment: Processes 1 and 2 are linked by a basolateral membrane Na-K-ATPase.

Type A intercalated cells

  1 Secrete hydrogen ions, which effect reabsorption of bicarbonate and excretion of titratable acid (stimulated by increased P_{CO_2} and decreased extracellular pH).

  2 Reabsorb potassium.

Comment: These 2 processes are linked by a luminal membrane H-K-ATPase.

Type B intercalated cells

  1 Reabsorb chloride (? stimulated by chloride depletion).

  2 Secrete bicarbonate (stimulated by increased extracellular pH).

Comment: These 2 processes are linked by a luminal membrane Cl-bicarbonate countertransporter.

* Functions of the inner medullary collecting-duct cells are not presented. Only the most important physiological regulators are given .

Appendix B

Table B–1. Classes of diurectics

Class	Mechanism	Major site affected
Carbonic anhydrase inhibitors	Inhibit secretion of hydrogen ions, which causes less reabsorption of bicarbonate and sodium	Proximal tubule
Loop diuretics	Inhibit Na, K, 2Cl cotransporter in luminal membrane	Thick ascending limb of Henle's loop
Thiazides	Inhibit Na, Cl cotransporter in luminal membrane	Distal convoluted tubule
Potassium-sparing diuretics*	Inhibit action of aldosterone	Cortical collecting duct
	Block sodium channels in luminal membrane	Collecting-duct system

* Except for this category, diuretics increase potassium excretion as well as sodium excretion (see text for discussion of the reasons for this increase). Aldosterone antagonists do not increase potassium excretion because they inhibit aldosterone's stimulation of potassium secretion. The sodium channel blockers also inhibit potassium secretion, in this case by reducing the amount of sodium entering the collecting duct cell for transport across the basolateral membrane by the Na-K-ATPase pumps; this reduces the activity of the pumps and, hence, the active transport of potassium into the cell.

Index

Page numbers followed by f and t indicate figures and tables, respectively.

205